To Thine Own "Health" Be True

Creating a Happier and Healthier

version of yourself

Let the Adventure Begin!

By

John Wilkins

ISBN-19: 9781798790526

Dedication

to Tim La Monte and Gene Hudson

"Friends who challenge and inspire"

And to the millions of people who are suffering needlessly from chronic diseases – this book is for you.

Table of Contents

Preface

I'm not a doctor or a health-care professional. I'm simply someone who was sick and was getting sicker while taking numerous prescription medications. I woke up one day and said, "Enough!" I subsequently spent months doing research and found what I believed were good sound principles that could lead me back to health. I followed the basic protocol of living a whole-food, plant-based lifestyle and in just 8 short weeks I turned my health completely around. I was healed of all my conditions and no longer needed the prescription meds I was taking. The tremendous and almost instantaneous results I achieved from changing my concept of "food" were so profound — **bordering on the miraculous** — that I was compelled to share my story with my friends and family, and ultimately with anyone else interested in taking control of their own health and healing. This book is anecdotal in nature and is simply one of thousands of personal stories demonstrating the amazing power of food as medicine. Much of the focus is on the personal struggle I experienced and how I found the motivation needed to succeed.

I'm personally indebted to the many people who have gone before me and shared their wisdom in documentaries, books, YouTube testimonials and Ted Talks. I have benefited greatly from their stories and research and I'm hoping this book will carry on the tradition of lifting others up, from ignorance and poor health situations, into the light and knowledge of vibrant health.

Subsequent to my illness and recovery, I formed the non-profit www.ourpassionforhealth.org, which is dedicated to educating and supporting those people who, like myself, are "sick and tired of being sick and tired" and want to reclaim their health once and for all. You are not in this alone! www.ourpassionforhealth.org wants you to be successful in finding your own path to a new life of energy and vitality. Life is a journey and that journey starts with a healthy body. Join the enlightened vanguard of living testimonials who are changing the way we think of food and ultimately how we think of our health.
Let the adventure begin! Let's change the world together, one bite at a time.

John Wilkins
March 21, 2019
Long Beach, Washington

INTRODUCTION

When asked what surprised him the most about humanity the Dalai Lama answered, "We sacrifice our health to gain wealth and then we spend all our wealth in order regain our health."

2018 marked the 100th anniversary of the great **influenza pandemic** of 1918. Between 50 and 100 million people are thought to have died, representing as much as 5 percent of the world's population. There were an estimated 675,000 flu deaths in America that year before it burned itself out. The whole country panicked lived in fear that they would be its next victim. As horrendous as that was, today, over 900,000 Americans die every year of chronic diseases, but no one is running around in fear for their lives. The big difference between these two great pandemics is that in 1918, there was nothing people could do to protect themselves (except quarantine) from the uncontrollable highly contagious flu virus.

The present health crisis is totally different. There is no run-away contagion. America's on-going poor health and resulting premature deaths are self-induced. In 1918 the pandemic attacked and killed innocent victims who had little control over the root infection. Today's victims, however, are not innocent and are, in fact, ultimately responsible for making the poor lifestyle choices that are making them sick. Millions are willfully feasting on poisons that they gladly consume. It's sad because today's victims don't see their personal health crisis coming until it's too late and they become a statistic.

How did this happen? Many researchers point to the fact that our eating habits are controlled and manipulated by clever, highly funded ads and propaganda campaigns designed to create cravings and addictions to *food-like* substances that are devoid of the nutrition the body needs. These powerful processed food manufacturers are clearly winning the war for the hearts, minds and stomachs of our citizens. How? Massive advertising, and they literally have no competition in this arena. There is no other opponent in the ring and there is virtually no push-back in terms of mass marketing and because of this lack, the citizens rarely see or hear a different point of view. The fast food industry spends over $4 billion dollars a year advertising their high calorie low nutrition products. When was the last time you noticed a TV commercial touting the benefits of eating a fresh and nutritious salad? Never! As a result, the deck is stacked against us. The fast food industries have succeeded in milking us for billions of dollars in profits while creating, on a mass scale, disease and chronic illness of every sort.

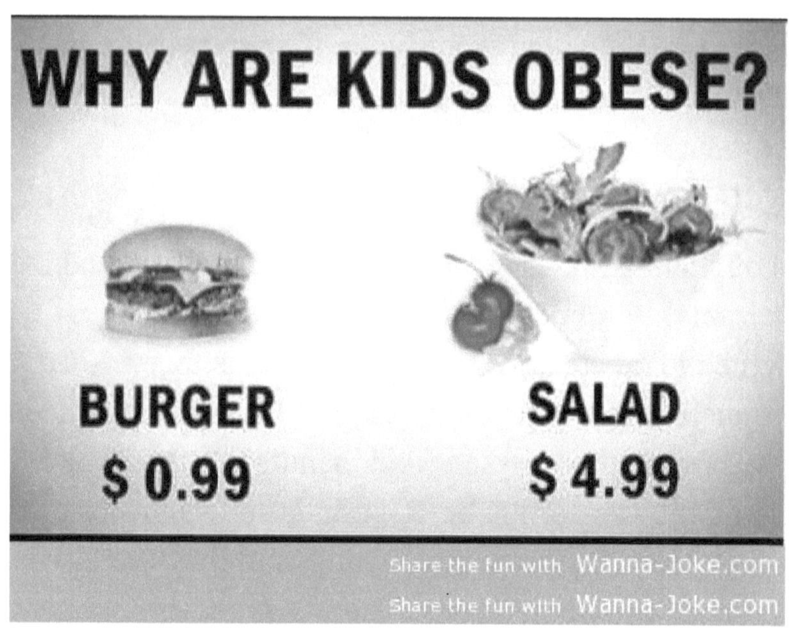

Just in case you are unaware of the extent of the current American Health Crisis, below are a few statistics and a list of our worst American epidemics.

Autoimmune Epidemic

Autoimmune Diseases — an epidemic bigger than cancer and heart disease combined! It's an epidemic affecting approximately 50 million Americans or 20% of the population (according to the National Institute of Health). Between 2000 and 2030, the number of Americans living with chronic disease is predicted to *increase* prevalence of autoimmune disease on the rise, more children *by 37%*. That is bad but here's the really upsetting part, with the are getting sick . . . and at a faster rate. In fact, autoimmune disease is one of the top 10 causes of death for kids aged 1–14 and one of the top 8 for all Americans.

Obesity Epidemic

An estimated 160 million Americans are either obese or overweight (that's almost half of all Americans!) Nearly three-quarters of American men, and more than **60%** of women, are obese or overweight and research has proven time and time again that being overweight leads to all sorts of physical ailments.

Diabetes Epidemic

In 2015, an estimated 1.5 million new cases of diabetes were diagnosed among people aged 18 and older. A new report from the US Centers for Disease Control and Prevention shows that *the number of Americans with diabetes continues to rise, with an estimated 12% of the adult population being diabetic.*

New CDC report: More than 100 million Americans have diabetes or prediabetes, and that's almost a third of all Americans.

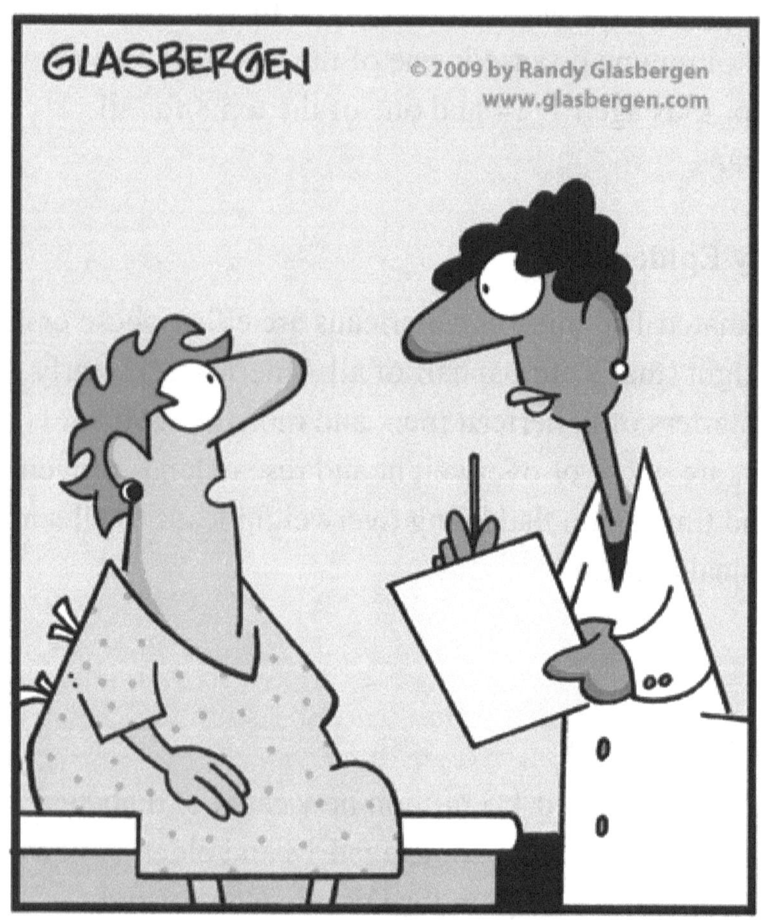

"I think diabetes is affecting my eyesight. I have trouble seeing the consequences of poor food choices."

Heart Disease Epidemic

New statistics predict that 45 percent of people in the United States will have at least one issue related to heart disease by 2035. The AHA predicts that costs related to the disease will double from $555 billion in 2016 to $1.1 trillion in 2035.

Financial Costs and Crisis

That "could bankrupt our nation's economy and healthcare system," according to AHA President Steven Houser, PhD.

About 610,000 people die of heart disease in the United States every year — that's 1 in every 4 deaths. Heart disease is the leading cause of death for both men and women.

A summary of the financial costs of the epidemics plaguing our country:

- $327 billion: Total costs of diagnosed diabetes in the United States in 2017
- Cost of Autoimmune Disease: estimated a total US cost of $112 Billion in 2013.
- costs related to Heart disease estimated at $555 billion in 2016
- That adds up to $994 Billion dollars today!
- That's almost a trillion dollars a year to treat Americans who could possibly heal themselves by making some lifestyle changes!!!

It Doesn't Have to be This Way!

Today, the vast majority of debilitating chronic diseases that lead ultimately to premature death could be totally avoided or reversed by Americans if they simply understood what it takes to keep the body healthy and happy. We are being foolish when we discount the value of a healthy body. Some would say that we are acting like fools when we continue to satisfy our food lusts and destructive cravings for manufactured food-like substances that have little nutritional value and are surely bringing us closer to our demise.

I too was addicted to sweet and salty food-like substances. I was captured by the sophisticated advertising and the naturally addictive nature of these "foods." I was guilty of willful ignorance regarding my diet and lifestyle. *Guilty!* I suffered for that ignorance for far too long. Fortunately for me, I woke up. Recognizing that something must be wrong if I'm forced to take four separate prescription medications for four different conditions. I became agitated and distressed with my unhealthy condition and this motivated me to start asking questions. I wanted honest and useful answers.

The answers I found were profound and I was so struck by the simplicity of the cure for my ailments, that I was compelled to share my story with those who, for whatever reason, aren't happy with the present condition of their health and want to return their bodies to a place of vitality.

This is also a cautionary tale for those who may be young and vital now and are wise enough to want to continue in good health for a lifetime.

Chapter 1

First Step: Let's Stop Taking Our Health for Granted!

Most of us would agree that absolutely nothing is more important than our overall health and wellbeing. It's hard to enjoy life if we are in pain or lack energy and vitality.

Even though we intuitively know this, many of us live our lives as though our health is the last thing on our minds. Like many good things in life, we take our health for granted, believing our questionable lifestyle and careless behavior will never catch up to us. This is partially due to the fact that our bodies are truly amazing in their efficiency and ability to repair and maintain themselves. This happens without us being aware of the internal healing process that goes on below our conscious mind. There are untold numbers of daily battles going on inside of us. The beneficial bacteria are trying to overcome the harmful bacteria, our white blood cells are cleaning up infections that are attacking etc. etc. Most of the time our bodies win the battles and the wars, but we are totally unaware of any of it . . . until the tide turns and we become sick. Then, if you are like me, you become impatient with the fact you are no longer feeling great, as though your body doesn't have the right to get sick and let you down. I understand. Personally, I hate it when I get a simple cold with the constant nose blowing, coughing, feverish weakness! I greatly appreciate it when I'm feeling better again and then, almost immediately, I go back to my daily routine and forget all about my body's health, taking it totally for granted once more.

What's the problem? We're eating garbage! (Remember the saying, "Garbage in = garbage out.") When it comes to our health, we're conflicted. American's are blessed to have the entire world of foods and tastes to choose from. When we ask ourselves, "What do I feel like eating today?" What we're really asking is, "What food am I craving today?" Do we choose the *taste* we want right now, or will we choose the *nutrient-filled foods* that build us up for tomorrow? Unfortunately, for millions of people the answer is right in front of them — the proliferation of fast food restaurants in every town across America answers that question.

How is it that we live in a country where the truth about health and nutrition is as easily available as a key stroke on the computer while most of us ignore and even shun the truth that could set us free from pain, sickness and suffering? Why aren't people interested in being healthy until they get sick? Could the problem have something to do with the old saying, "If it's not broke, don't fix it?" The crazy thing is that even when people do contract a chronic disease, and it's obvious to all that their body is broken, they still won't do what is necessary to fix it. Most of us will ignorantly take prescription drugs to mask the symptoms of the disease, but will not make the lifestyle changes necessary to address the root cause, thus ridding themselves of the disease completely and ultimately bringing their body back to vital health once again.

Fortunately, our bodies are powerful physical machines. It may take many years before we see the results of bad lifestyle choices. However, when we do start to feel the effects, it may be too late. The good news is that it is possible to change course and snap back and not only regain our previous level of health but surpass it and feel more vital than ever before. I know this is possible because it happened to me.

I'm a typical Baby-Boomer. Sure, I'm getting up in age and I can accept that, but what I don't like is the fact that I'm not as strong as I once was. I've gotten progressively weaker and put on some pounds. In the meantime, I've developed high blood pressure combined with high blood sugar. I have stomach problems — gastroesophageal reflux disease — plus I have an enlarged prostate. I put up with these slight health deficiencies with a stiff upper lip AND with the usual prescription drugs that masked all the symptoms. *I'm aging, but no big deal, that's life,* I thought, and I was able to ignore what was happening to me until I reached a point where I had a serious health crisis.

Getting sick was strange to me because I've always been relatively healthy. I'd get a cold once a year and that was about it. I've been physically active all my life. I played sports in my youth and played tennis, surfed and snow skied as an adult. So, I was generally healthy and in good shape for the most part and I never really gave my eating and drinking habits any thought at all.

Then, all of a sudden, I was "awakened" and shaken to the core by an illness, Polymyalgia Rheumatica (PMR), a crippling autoimmune disease that attacks the large muscles and joints. I went from taking a serious mountain biking trip one day to being crippled the next! Seriously, I needed to bend over to walk, looking and feeling like an old man. In addition, I couldn't raise my arms above my head making it almost impossible to wash or comb my hair. That got my attention! I was devastated and honestly frightened at what was happening to my body. I'll never forget the day I woke up with an overwhelming sense of dread and I began to contemplate how I could end my life of pain. I just couldn't imagine living my remaining years in a body that was broken and almost useless. But sometimes good things can come from bad circumstances and so it was in my case. Fortunately, I had a few close friends to talk to who encouraged me and gave me hope.

One was Aunt Ruthie who happened to be a wise, 87-year-old nutritionist.

I can say, without a doubt, the autoimmune disease, PMR scared the bad lifestyle out of me. It woke me up and Ruthie gave me a new vision for my health that was actually exciting. My life changed when I began to take my health seriously, meaning, I took the time and effort to get educated. As a result of questioning and searching and probing what it means to be "healthy", I found out that *it is possible to turn back time*, and become vital again, even in my 60's. My desperate search lead to the answers that helped me to overcome my deteriorating health. Those answers were simple and yet profound, and to my amazement, they worked!

Based on my research, I know that there are millions of Americans suffering from various chronic diseases and are forced to take prescription drugs to mask their symptoms. I now believe that the vast majority of those people can turn the tide and get back to robust health and off most, if not all, their prescription medications by learning what I learned over the past year. I promise you, there is a better way!

Too many Americans are caught up in the American Health Care System, a system that, in partnership with the pharmaceutical industry, treats the symptoms of disease and not the disease itself. This is the primary problem with our current health care system and this needs to change, starting with me and you.

Chapter 2

How Could This Happen to Me?

For some, illness and disease may come on quickly but for most, it's a gradual thing. For me it started with heartburn. I ate hot and spicy foods for years with no problems or repercussions. Indian food was one of my favorites. Butter Chicken called to me once a week. I had consistent cravings for Thai and Chinese food, pizza, ice cream, buttered popcorn and alcohol etc. etc. You get the idea. I liked to eat and drink what I wanted when I wanted. From time to time I was truly glutenous, like that time I ate two, back-to-back steak and lobster dinners followed by coffee, cheese cake and chocolate mousse. I was on a cruise ship (obviously) and was up all night feeling miserable and hating myself for being so stupid. I spent some time the next day writing in my journal about the sin of gluttony.

Fortunately, I had a metabolism that burned up most of what I ate so I didn't get fat until I got into my 50s. All I noticed was, I was having a harder time getting into my pants. I put on a few pounds and bought bigger pants and longer belts. *No problem. No big deal. This was expected at my age, right?* But then I began to get occasional heartburn. I'd take Tums or Rolaids to stop the burning and go about my business. Soon I had to have the tums in my pocket when I left the house just to be prepared for the heartburn when it came, and it came a lot. Eventually, the heartburn became so frequent, almost daily, that my doctor prescribed Prilosec, (**omeprazole**) is a **proton pump inhibitor** that decreases the amount of acid produced in the stomach. Prilosec worked great and I began to take it daily. The heartburn stopped, and I could eat anything I wanted to, any time. This was fantastic! No problems. But, of course, there was a problem. On the box it says to take Prilosec for only 28 days unless your doctor tells you otherwise. So, after taking the pill every day for 3 years I went to my gastroenterologist to ask him about the possible side effects. He said there were a few but that in his opinion, "getting rid of the heartburn was worth it. The side effects were less troubling than the heartburn itself, so keep taking the pills". Recently I looked up the possible side effects of prolonged use of Prilosec.

The Side Effects of Prilosec

- severe stomach pain, diarrhea that is watery or bloody;
- a rash or joint pain;
- new or unusual pain in your wrist, thigh, hip, or back;

- seizure (convulsions);
- kidney problems — urinating more or less than usual, blood in your urine, swelling, rapid weight gain;
- symptoms of low magnesium — drowsiness, confusion, feeling irritable, fast heartbeats, tremors, twitching, muscle cramps, numbness, tingling, or seizure, stomach pain, gas;
- nausea, vomiting, diarrhea;
- headache;
- post-marketing reports: Anxiety, apathy, nervousness, dream abnormalities, psychiatric and sleep disturbances[Ref]
- Confusion, agitation, aggression, depression, and hallucinations occurring predominantly in severely ill or elderly patients.[Ref]

This is not a complete list of side effects and others may occur.

So there you have it! I was feeling some pain in my joints and I might have had more problems associated with Prilosec, but I ignored them. The point is that my doctor never mentioned that it might be a good idea to examine what I was eating, or to change my diet and heal my gut and be rid of the problem once and for all. There was absolutely no discussion about alternatives to taking Prilosec, nor any hint given that it's possible to recover and be healed from the disease. **The current medical**

profession is trained to treat the symptoms of disease and not to heal the disease itself. So, I left his office feeling like Prilosec was a part of my daily routine and I continued to take the pills for another 3 years before I got really sick and was forced to make some changes.

In the meantime, I noticed that my blood pressure was going up a little more each time I had occasion to take it at the doctor's office. It took a few years for the blood pressure to approach levels that are considered "high" for my height and weight, but my doctor never mentioned it or brought it up. It was my sister who became alarmed when she found out what my blood pressure was (170 over 100). She was a *wanna-be* nurse. She was a licensed phlebotomist and her dad, my step-dad, was an MD and she worked in his office for years and eventually went to nursing school, so she was knowledgeable. She begged me to get medication to bring down the blood pressure because, as she said, "It's not about the heart attack. It's about the stroke that will leave you paralyzed and in a wheel chair for the rest of your life." That sounded scary to me, and the next time I went for my annual physical I asked my doctor what she thought, and she agreed with my sister and put me on 10mg of Lisinopril. **Lisinopril** is an ACE inhibitor. ACE stands for angiotensin converting enzyme. Lisinopril is used to treat high blood pressure (hypertension) in adults and it worked. My blood pressure went from an average of 170 over 100 to 135 over 80. Again, there was no discussion with my doctor about what

I was doing or eating or drinking that might affect my blood pressure. There were no suggestions about making diet or lifestyle changes that might correct the problem and bring the high blood pressure down to a safe level WITHOUT taking the drug. And of course, there was no talk about the side effects of taking the drug. None at all.

The Side Effects of Lisinopril

- blurred vision
- cloudy urine
- confusion
- decrease in urine output or decrease in urine-concentrating ability
- dizziness, faintness, or lightheadedness when getting up suddenly from a lying or sitting position
- sweating
- unusual tiredness or weakness
- Abdominal or stomach pain
- body aches or pain
- chest pain
- chills
- common cold
- cough
- diarrhea
- difficulty breathing
- ear congestion
- fever
- headache

- loss of voice
- nasal congestion
- nausea
- runny nose
- sneezing
- sore throat
- vomiting
- decreased interest in sexual intercourse
- inability to have or keep an erection
- lack or loss of strength
- loss in sexual ability, desire, drive, or performance
- rash
- acid or sour stomach
- belching
- burning, crawling, itching, numbness, prickling, pins and needles, or tingling feelings
- feeling of constant movement of self or surroundings
- heartburn
- indigestion
- muscle cramps
- sensation of spinning
- stomach discomfort or upset
- swelling

Considering all the possible side effects, it might have been prudent to come up with an alternative to taking the drug.

When I started taking Lisinopril, I immediately felt a little dizzy and weak, like my blood had thinned out. I didn't feel like myself. I lacked energy and I stopped taking the pills. A year later after reading an article about high blood pressure, I found the pills and started taking them again, this time with no noticeable affects.

Of course, I do understand that if one has high blood pressure that is currently in the danger zone, taking a pill once a day to bring it down to a safe level makes sense on a "first-aid emergency" basis. However, I think there should have been some discussion about what caused this condition in the first place and what natural course of action I might take to remedy the problem. Don't you think?

So, I'm on two medications now that have a litany of possible side effects, but, I'm OK with it all because I'm trusting my doctors. They know best, right? Basically, I don't know any better, just like the people in the 18th century who listened to their doctors and allowed them to use blood sucking leaches to "bleed out" their sickness and disease. (I'm not making this up!)

At this point, I'm in no pain. I can eat and drink what I want with no apparent repercussions . . . and that's the problem. For most people, including myself, if one isn't experiencing any discomfort then there just doesn't seem to be any impetus to change anything. Life goes on.

Everything seems good on the surface, on a conscious level. I'm doing what I've always done and I'm happy. I'm not alarmed by the fact that I'm taking prescription drugs loaded with side effects because I'm not aware of them. I don't notice any side effects at this point. Unfortunately, looking back, I was naive believing everything was OK going forward. No pain or discomfort, therefore I don't need to change anything, right?

About this time, I realized that I was getting up in the middle of the night to pee. Usually not a big deal, but when the frequency increased to three times a night, I knew something wasn't right. I went to a urologist, took some tests and sure enough, there was a problem. My prostate gland was enlarged which didn't allow my bladder to fully drain, thus creating the frequent urination situation. But of course, there was a pill for that too. My new doctor put me on Flomax, a drug that was supposed to solve the problem. **Flomax** (tamsulosin) is an alpha-blocker that relaxes the muscles in the prostate and bladder neck, making it easier to urinate. Flomax is used to improve urination in men with benign prostatic hyperplasia (enlarged prostate). And again, there are a few possible side effects.

Common Side Effects of Flomax

- dizziness
- lightheadedness

- weakness, drowsiness
- headache
- nausea
- diarrhea
- back pain
- blurred vision
- dental problems
- sleep problems (insomnia)
- abnormal ejaculation
- decreased sex drive
- runny or stuffy nose
- sore throat
- cough
- an erection that is painful or lasts more than four hours, (No, I never experienced this!)
- severe dizziness, or
- fainting.

My doctor never mentioned any of the above possible side effects except to say that when I ejaculated, my ejaculate might go inside and not outside of my penis, but that's not a big deal, right? So, I added that prescription drug to my daily regimen. One of the side effects not mentioned by my doctor was the possibility of severe dizziness and fainting.

A few months later, on an annual Big Sur camping trip with my surfing buddies, I fainted. We were eating breakfast at a local restaurant when I suddenly keeled over and passed out. I was just sitting there, and I felt the Sun shining on the right side of my face and I started getting light-headed. Then I felt all the energy draining out of my body and I lost control of my muscles and I couldn't sit up anymore. I was in a booth and I just fell over onto my left side. One of my camping friends was a doctor and he felt no pulse and called 911. By this time I was laying on the floor with my feet elevated. I eventually came to and called off the ambulance ride. I thought the fainting was a result of being dehydrated from the heavy campfire drinking the night before, but I didn't know for sure. I felt dizzy and faint a number of times over the next year. One time I went to the hospital after a particularly bad dizzy spell. They thought I'd had a transient ischemic attack, or in layman's terms, a mini-stroke but after a battery of tests, they couldn't find anything wrong with me. Interestingly, the doctors never made the connection between the drugs I was taking and the fainting spells, even though 2 of the 3 drugs I was currently taking listed fainting and dizziness as a side effect of the drug. Had I been tipped off then, I might have been motivated to find an alternative to taking the drugs . . . maybe.

Looking back, I felt bad because of the incredible waste of money spent on a trip to the emergency room and the battery of tests to search for a problem that may have been caused by following my doctor's orders — taking prescription drugs. At this point no one, including myself, made the connection. I was in the dark and still counting on my doctor's expertise to keep me going strong. Does this sound familiar to anyone?

About this time I had a serious bicycle accident. I didn't know if the drugs that caused the dizziness and blurred vision had anything to do with the accident or if it was the combination of the drugs and alcohol. The alcohol, for sure, was a factor and combined with the Flomax and the Lisinopril — both of which list dizziness and fainting as a side effect — it probably added to the possibility of a crash.

So, on this beautiful Saturday afternoon, I was out riding my e-bike (electric bike) with a friend. We rode around town visiting other friends who gave us beer and wine at each stop. On the way home, I was coming down a steep hill, hit some gravel on the side of the road and lost control of my bike. I went off the street, hit a ditch, went over the handle bars landing on my head and back. I woke up with a group of people standing over me including a fireman bending over my limp body. Evidently, I'd been knocked out cold for a few minutes. They wanted to take me to the hospital, but, being embarrassed and foolish, I refused . . . mostly because I didn't want to take a chance of getting a DUI! (Yes! You can get a DUI on a bike!) They checked me out for serious injury, saw that I was bleeding from the head and back, had gravel embedded in my eyebrow, and my left wrist was tender to the touch. Nevertheless, I insisted I was OK. Despite their efforts, they allowed me to walk my bike home, but only after I signed a detailed legal form that stated that I made the decision, on my own, not go to the hospital and they were therefore off the hook and not responsible for any injuries or complications that might ensue, including my possible death. I suffered for the next 24 hours before I realized my wrist was broken and the pain was telling me to go to the doctor. It turned out that I broke my wrist in two places and experienced a shoulder separation. I still had gravel imbedded in my back and eyebrow and in my skull and the doctor was helpful in picking the gravel out of my body. Just for the record, I want to express my appreciation to the doctor who was extremely helpful in treating my injuries. This is where the medical profession shines. Emergency medicine! Thank you, Dr. Brown.

The fact is, I was really lucky! There was a telephone pole only a few feet away and had I hit the pole, with no helmet on, I would have been really messed up. (I learned from my mistake and I now wear a helmet when riding my bike AND I never drink and ride (or drive) — ever!) I mention this only because looking back it was kind of cool going 45 mph down a steep hill on a bike at 69 years old, crash, refuse the ambulance and make it home on my own with all my injuries. It was stupid and foolish but a little macho and when you are 69 years old, a little macho goes aa long way. You need a little adventure story in your life once in a while to feel like a man. Just saying. And yes, I ran with the bulls in Pamplona Spain in the year 2002. Macho.

Now, with my newfound macho, I'm taking a new drug, a pain killer. I'm fortunate that I'm not the type that wants to be drugged. I like feeling alive and well and pain killers are not appealing to me. I don't want my senses to be deadened. I want to be up and experiencing life to the fullest. Opioids are dangerous and a downer and I'm not into that. That time was an example of taking a drug for an acute situation and no doubt, a pain killer is a God-send when you need it, but for me it was only a temporary need. I was off them in two days.

Chapter 3

The Final Straw

So, what happened next? It was very unfortunate, and I hesitate to even mention it, but it's honest and may have something to do with my next medical set back. After many years of marriage, my wife and I broke up. It's unfortunate, but let's just say our marriage had run its course. This was a lot harder on me than on her because she kept the house we had lived in the for 12 years. I had to move out and as we all know, moving is a major hassle filled with stress. I thought I'd be in that house for the rest of my life. I made the move, doing all the packing and sorting and went from a 4,000 sq. foot home overlooking the ocean to temporarily renting a room from a friend of mine across town. As you can imagine, the divorce and moving caused a lot of stress for me, and we all know that excess stress can be a killer.

About a month or so after I moved out, I went on a mountain bike ride with my friends. It was a grueling day of riding with a lot of pounding ruts on the path. Normally not a problem, but the next morning when I woke up I felt a pain in my left hip. I assumed it was a pulled muscle and didn't give it much thought at the time, but the next day when I woke up, the other hip was involved and hurting too. I knew immediately it was more than a pulled muscle, but still I wasn't too worried about it until the next day when I woke up and both my shoulders were hurting to the extent that I couldn't lift my arms above my head without excruciating pain.

At this point, I knew I had a serious problem. Each day my pain got worse. In two weeks' time, I was bent over like an old man just trying to walk. Needless to say, I went to my primary care physician. She didn't have a clue what was wrong with me. She told me to take ibuprofen for the pain, which I did for 60 days. The ibuprofen barely deadened the pain. I'm not one to take aspirin or pain killers of any type, but for two months I took 4 ibuprofen every four hours, day and night just to try to get by. During that time, I went on our annual men's trip, this time to Washington to climb mountains. Despite the handfuls of ibuprofen I took, I was lagging behind the group. I thought about quitting and turning back a number of times. I made it to the top eventually, but I wasn't my usual self and I was suffering constantly. Again, the macho thing — trying to prove I could still keep up with the younger guys in the group.

When I returned home, I immediately made an appointment with my doctor. When I saw her, I got a little aggressive. I said, "You are my primary care physician and I'm in excruciating pain and taking handfuls of ibuprofen day and night, which can't be good for me, and I can barely walk. What's going on with my body?! "She ordered some blood tests and when the results came back, she was able to correctly diagnose the problem. I had developed a crippling autoimmune disease called Polymyalgia Rheumatica (PMR).

Polymyalgia Rheumatica results from an overabundance of inflammation in one's system, which causes widespread aching and stiffness in one's large joints and muscles. Symptoms tend to come on quickly, over a few days or weeks, and sometimes even overnight. Both sides of the body are equally affected. Involvement of the upper arms, with trouble raising them above the shoulders, is common. Sometimes, aching occurs at joints such as the hips, hands and wrists. I had all of the symptoms in spades. It's a terribly painful and crippling disease.

Needless to say, this illness was different. For the first time in my life, I experienced gut-wrenching pain that wouldn't go away on its own. Suddenly, I was paying attention to my body and my body was screaming out loud, "I'm mad as hell and I'm not going to take it anymore!"* (From the great movie, *Network*.)

The good news and the bad news is that the doctors have a remedy for this ailment too: the powerful and fast acting prescription steroidal drug called "prednisone." Steroid drugs, such as prednisone, work by lowering the activity of the immune system. The immune system is your body's defense system. Steroids work by slowing your body's response to disease or injury. (Sounds great, doesn't it?!) Prednisone can help lower certain immune-related symptoms, including inflammation and swelling, but it's a mixed bag. It lowers your body's ability to fight off disease AND it also lowers the inflammation and stops the pain! I was thinking, *It can Stop the pain? Then bring it on immediately, NOW please!* (At that point I was not macho . . . not at all. All I cared about was stopping the pain.) Once again the doctors focused on the symptoms and, in this case, I wanted the symptoms to go away, so all was well. When I took the prednisone, I noted six hours later that the pain had subsided. I was experiencing my first pain-free moment in 3 months. It was almost a miracle to me at the time. When someone has a boot on your throat for months and then takes it off, it feels great to be boot free and pain free for a change. So, I give credit to the pharmaceutical company that perfected this cortical steroid that relieves pain. But of course, like most drugs, Prednisone has its dark side . . . the bad news:

The Many Side Effects of Prednisone:
- confusion

- excitement
- restlessness
- headache
- nausea
- vomiting
- thinning skin
- acne
- trouble sleeping
- weight gain
- Severe allergic reactions
- Changes in emotions or moods, such as depression
- Changes in vision
- Eye pain
- Infection. Symptoms can include:
  - fever or chills
  - cough
  - sore throat
  - trouble or pain in passing urine
- High blood sugar with symptoms of:
  - increased thirst
  - passing urine more often
  - feeling sleepy or confused
  - swelling of your ankles or feet

There are more, but I think you get the idea. Getting rid of the pain with prednisone is like making a deal with the devil and I had to make that deal, at least for the time being.

So, now I'm on 4 prescription medications that all have side effects of some kind. Of course, it's important to understand that there is always a tradeoff. Ask yourself, *Are the side effects worse than the disease or the symptoms it eliminates? Are you willing to take a chance? What are the odds?* I believe it's OK to take prescription drugs for a short time. You have a health issue. This might be a good time to assess the problem, determine what caused it and maybe learn how you can reverse this negative trend and ultimately become healthy again and get off all the drugs. I now look at the need for a prescription drug as a wakeup call and taking the drug as "first-aid", but you don't want to make it the long-term solution. The faster you can get off the synthetic drug substances the better. I realize this now, but I didn't back then.

Chapter 4

Revelation!

A change was coming. A month after being introduced to prednisone, I was mostly pain free and I took a trip to La Paz Mexico to visit my sister who had moved there a few years earlier. While there, I had time to relax and think about my worsening health crisis. In the weeks prior to this visit, I watched a few Netflix health-oriented documentaries and Ted Talks. I was looking for answers to my newest problem, Polymyalgia Rheumatica (PMR), the autoimmune disease. This setback was my personal wake up call. The pain and suffering I experienced with PMR got my attention like nothing else could. I was sincerely frightened, not knowing if I'd be able to be well and 100% healthy again. I was in my sixties. Was my life over? Had I reached the point of no return? No! I loved life and I couldn't and wouldn't accept that. I liked being physically active, which was no problem with the other ailments I was treating with drugs, but this was different. For me it wasn't just the pain, it was the idea that the pain was so severe that I couldn't be myself . . . my physically active self. By now I had dropped out of the tennis club, I stopped playing golf, I couldn't surf anymore because my shoulders hurt so much, I simply couldn't paddle my surfboard. This fact made me miserable. Regardless, I wasn't going down without a fight.

I did some checking around and I discovered that the only effective drug for PMR was prednisone, and though very effective in relieving the pain, it had one of the longest lists of side effects in the pharmaceutical world. I didn't want to be on this drug any longer than necessary and I was seriously looking for answers, and for me that meant taking a deep dive into the medical research and then into the world of holistic healing. Holistic healing? Desperate people will do desperate things.

While I was relaxing in Mexico, I began to mentally review various health strategies I'd picked up while studying over the previous month. The ideas that made the most sense to me were mostly restorative in nature. I was thinking about partial fasting, juice rebooting, yoga, meditation (to lower blood pressure) followed by what looked like a more restrictive approach — embracing dramatic lifestyle changes. *Could it be that all the body needs is the right fuel to supply the proper nutrients and vitamins and building blocks necessary to restore health and become vital again?*

That's what I was thinking about as I sat in my lounge chair by the pool. Despite the pristine ocean view, it was depressing to think about my predicament. Something needed to change, and I became totally obsessed with the idea of getting well. I wanted to be young again, I wanted to be active again, I wanted to be myself again! This single-minded focus led me to what I'll call a "personal revelation". I experienced a very clear thought that led to an idea and when I subsequently embraced the idea it produced innate POWER!

What if I could use my body as a science experiment? I'd watched enough health documentaries to know there were answers out there. That was the problem. There were so many different ways to go on this health journey, where was I supposed to start? What if I tried these various avenues until I found one solid direction that worked for me and then I could document my experience and add it to the others.

I was excited. This seemed like a good way to spend my retirement years. I could help myself and help others in the process. That was the exact moment I was turned on to the idea of chasing "Uber Health". My vision of being on a quest for health restoration energized me and gave me hope. I would dedicate the rest of my life to finding answers that would put me into a place I'd never been before health wise. I'd learn what to do to get healthy and I'd do it no matter how hard or seemingly sacrificial the journey might be.

Here is my basic idea and vision: I would find the answers, turn my health around in a dramatic fashion, and show others how to do the same. That's it. It was a good idea and a worthy goal.

THE HARD PART: For me, taking the leap of faith to be committed 100% to the best health possible, and being willing to do whatever was necessary to get there, was - by far - the most difficult part. I had to continually talk myself into crossing that bridge. It was like jumping off the high diving board for the first time when I was a kid. I wanted to do it, others proved it could be done and were doing it and encouraging me to do it, but I was afraid to jump. But when I finally got the guts to take that leap, it all worked out and I was very proud of myself for doing it. Now, as an adult, I'm afraid I'll fail if I try to radically change my diet and lifestyle. I didn't know if I could do it. I tried to shift my focus away from what I might have to give up and onto the way I'd feel about being ultimately successful. It wasn't going to be easy and I knew instinctively that the price I'd have to pay to find out, was for me, a big price. No more beer, sweets and maybe no red meat? So, I used logic, reason, and creative philosophy to urge me forward. I continually reminded myself of the righteous truth and wisdom that was associated with my goal. No doubt, getting back my health, whatever the cost, would certainly be worth it. I think we can all agree with that, right?

A lot of what I've shared in this book is about this critical part: believing **it's worth the effort** and believing you can do it. To get there you'll need to find good reasons why making the change is the best decision you could possibly make at this specific point in your life. This is why your personal search is so important. You need to get up to speed and understand that this decision is profound and meaningful in all the right ways. I promise you this, if you seek out the truth concerning your health, you will find what you are looking for and then you'll have the inner power to make the change. The more you know, the stronger your resolve. Like the Bible says: "the truth will set you free."

The critical starting point for change is knowing and understanding deep in your heart and soul that there is absolutely and positively nothing more important in your entire life than obtaining and maintaining your good health! It doesn't matter how many homes you own or how much money you have, if you don't have your health, life can suck. Despite this fact, a fact that we may not have come to terms with yet, as previously pointed out, we continually take our health for granted. Our bodies are so well made that we can abuse them for years and years before the body says *enough!* Eventually our body breaks down and we are no longer at ease and we now are experiencing dis-ease.

But I've learned that disease is not necessary, even later in life. Untold numbers of books and documentaries tell us that our bodies are amazing and resilient. With proper care and feeding we can recover and come back to being strong, healthy and vital again. You need to believe this!

Based on what I had gleaned at that point, I came to believe that I could reverse the damage I'd done to my body and literally turn back time regarding my health. My vision and goal in life now was to continue my study. I was using the internet, watching health documentaries, reading health and diet books and formulating a master plan that would accomplish my goal which was to be off all my prescription medications and be as healthy as possible in the next six months. If I could accomplish this goal, I'll have proven the power of innate health over drugs. It's the difference between:

a) taking control of your health and choosing to be well, or
b) ignorantly taking prescription drugs designed to diminish the symptoms of the disease (and not addressing the root causes) while your core health deteriorates.

I was hoping my personal breakthrough would give hope and inspiration to others who are aware and ready to make a change. This is about waking up, becoming educated, and understanding what true health is and how to regain it and personally maintain it. I told myself:

- If I must fast, I'll fast
- If I must stop drinking alcohol, I'll stop
- If I must stop eating red meat, I'll stop

- No more sugar or breads, I'll do it
- And If I must eat only vegetables and fruit, I'll do that and anything else because I believe *IT WILL BE WORTH IT!*

I decided finally that I'd do whatever it takes! I'd try one thing after another and then a combination of things until I found the answers that worked for me. And, I decided to document the journey step by step. My goal would be to share the details with others, demonstrating how they too can recover their health, should that, someday become a priority for them. I finally sold myself on the idea. I was energized and motivated to the max. I couldn't wait to get back to Santa Cruz and get started.

When I left Mexico I was a new man. I went there with a heavy heart, physically and mentally drained and depressed. I had no vision, and as the Bible says: "Without a vision, the people perish." and I was perishing, but now, everything seemed different.

It's been said, "The most powerful thing in the world is an idea whose time has come". I think it's helpful to personalize this with a statement of commitment and strength:

> *Right now there is nothing more powerful nor more important for me than to embrace this healthy lifestyle. It's now my number 1. priority. There is power in a*

*good idea and I'm feeling this
power now!*

I boarded the plane for home with a clear vision. I was
energized and looking forward to my new life of
exploration and purpose. When I arrived home, I'd start
immediately. I was now on a mission to repair my body
and become physically active once again. I was feeling
great and fully alive and I was very happy and excited
about the new life that was before me.

It must be repeated: you need to embrace the idea that
there is nothing more important than your health. Think
about it. Do you put your kids above your health? You
shouldn't because if you aren't healthy and vital how can
you properly serve your children in the best possible way?
And for spiritually minded people who want to put God
first, ahead of your health somehow? I'd say, let's
remember, God (Nature, the Universe) gave you an
amazing gift — your physical body — and expects you to
respect and cherish that gift because it's what and who you
are Christians! According to the Bible, your body is very
important:

1 Corinthians 6:19–20

[19]"Do you not know that your
bodies are temples of the Holy
Spirit, who is in you, whom you
have received from God?

<blockquote>Therefore, honor God with your bodies."</blockquote>

Your body is the temple of God! And that would indicate that God wants his temple to be taken care of in the best possible way. So, if you love God, demonstrate that love by taking care of his temple, right? For any atheists that may be reading this, just embrace the idea that your body is you and if you care about yourself and your life, then care about your body and its health.

Key point: this idea and vision, that so dramatically changed my life for good, came about because I was motivated to find the truth regarding my health. The more I searched, the more I found and what I found seemed well substantiated and documented to the point where I believed that what I was learning was true. I believed, if I moved forward in the right direction, I'd be healed. To make that happen, I needed to continue my education. I found that it helped immensely to observe others who had gone before me. I'm very thankful that many were willing to share their personal experiences with me. I watched dozens of YouTube videos of people who had traveled this road before me and were successful and happy to share the details of how they did it. I believed if they could do it, I could do it. Like them, I could choose the "path least traveled" and I could be restored to excellent health too. It does take a leap of faith and you need to get to that place where you know enough and feel comfortable enough to make the leap.

There is little hope in being successful in this health journey until you are convinced in your mind and soul that you know what you are doing and why, and you know ultimately that it's going to be worth it.

Chapter 5

The Plan

Once home, I immediately dove into my research to find the right starting path to ultimate health. This wasn't as easy as it sounds. I'm sure you are aware that there are many health diets and modalities and theories and supplements all competing for our attention. I didn't want to go through a hit or miss period for a prolonged time. I wanted to zero in on a few ideas that looked reasonable and promising. My first thought was, I'd try the easiest "fix" and move toward more radical lifestyle changes later if necessary.

First, I reviewed my goals, which were twofold:

1. To find a path to superior and vibrant health, thus reaching a point where I am prescription drug free.
2. To document my journey in book and possibly film so other likeminded people might benefit from the positive experience I was anticipating.

Now that I had a good understanding of what I was destined to do, I jumped in with both feet and focused my brain. I spent all my days and nights reading books, listening to podcasts, watching documentaries, Ted Talks and YouTube testimonials . . . and I loved every minute of it!

I felt like I was trying to solve a riddle or a puzzle as complex as the universe, but I was undaunted. I could look for clues anywhere and everywhere. During this time I saw the world through the eyes of a man on a mission. As I looked around, I started to notice the large number of obese people everywhere. I thought of the concept of being fat myself, which I was, but didn't realize it then. Let's just say I wasn't technically obese; my number didn't hit that part of the scale, but I was getting close.

As I looked for specific answers to specific questions, I realized that I was getting a little obsessed with the whole idea of what I was doing, but I think it's a good idea to become obsessed about being healthy and I never strayed from my focus. I made it my life's mission and I had a single-minded attention to one thing . . . *uber health!* Now in "scholar mode" my research led me to a clear perception of what the latest scientific ideas were regarding our understanding of the human body and how it works best.

While studying I was encouraged to find that there is a radical movement in the field of medicine. There are now "functional doctors." These are MDs who are all about the holistic approach to medicine. They start with the idea that our bodies were meant to be and to stay healthy. Sickness is not the norm, health is. And when someone comes into the doctor's office with a pain, the "functional doctor" takes the time to find out what the underlying root cause of the pain is and then the doctor can come up with a plan to rid the patient of the pain or ailment once and for all. I was fortunate to find Dr. Jay Pennock, a functional doctor who provided great support for my journey. Our country has 99% traditional doctors. That's the problem. The solution is functional doctors. There is a visionary in the field and he's written a book I would highly recommend. It should be "must reading" for all Medical School freshmen. It's called *The Evolution of Medicine* by James Maskell. Check it out!

At this point, I'm a curious sponge soaking up interesting, cutting-edge information about the nature of health. There is a powerful truth about our health that I came to know and that every human being should be aware of and master. Yes, I said "master"! I sincerely believe it is our individual responsibility as human beings to know the basics of how our body works and how we can best maintain and nourish it. Doesn't that make sense?

We all complain that our medical insurance costs too much. Why do you think that is? It's obvious. It's because too many Americans are sick with chronic illnesses and diseases and the medical establishment is doing very little to heal those diseases. They make more money by keeping us in a perpetual state of *dis-ease* where we have to keep coming back to be monitored and get our next prescription drug. It's called the "Medical Industrial Complex" and it's got to change. We want to go to a place in the future where eating smart is common knowledge, even among the barely educated, meaning everyone will know instinctively that paying attention to one's health should be life's number one priority. What could be more important than that? This is not selfish. There is nothing more altruistic than taking care of yourself first, so you can then be in a strong position to help others.

You are going to need motivation and here is a thought. If you say you want more energy in your life, then what you really want is to experience a higher degree of health because when you are eating nutritious foods, with all their inherent vitamins and minerals, the body responds with added reserves of energy, compared to eating at McDonalds. To be your best is to be your healthiest. To be your smartest is to be your healthiest!

(Philosophical comment coming . . .) Being *Uber Healthy* It's the least you can do to show your appreciation for being given such a great gift: a human body on planet earth. Think about it! As far as we know, the greatest thing in the universe is to be a "conscious human being" and to be able to live a full and rich life. You are like a child of God (of the universe, of the creative substance, whatever your idea of the life force is . . .), AND you are literally made of stardust! The elements you are made up of were created at the center of an exploding star. How cool is that! You are part of the ultimate drama of the Universe created by an all-mighty power that we can only attempt to imagine . . . but can't possibly. Never forget, your life is an amazing gift filled with wonder, drama and adventure! All I'm saying is, please appreciate this fact. Gratitude, wonder and appreciation for your life are the first steps on the road to healthy living. The way it works is all so fantastic . . . treat your body and your life with respect and in a way that shows your appreciation for being one of the chosen few. Be happy and enjoy your wonderful existence. Every second you are alive is a miracle. Mathematician and astrophysicist, Ben Carney, puts it this way,

> "There is 1 chance in 140 trillion that the
> Earth should exist. There is 1 chance in 795
> billion that life should have evolved on earth.
> There is 1 chance in 89 billion that life should
> have evolved into mankind. There is 1 chance
> in 12 billion that mankind should have created
> the alphabet and thus civilization. There is 1
> chance in 6 billion that your parents should
> ever have met and got together. There is 1
> chance in 90 million that you should have
> been the lucky sperm that fertilized your
> mother's egg . You have won the cosmic
> lottery!"

Like I said, you and your life on earth are special. Your direct connection to this experience is through the five senses of your physical body so it makes *sense* to take good care of it, right?

My Core Belief:

> *Nothing is more self-empowering than taking control of one's health. It creates inner power AND good health. This is such a great truth! Anyone in America, no matter how poor or weak or socially marginalized, can transform their lives for the better by simply taking control of what they put into their mouths each day. You can buck the trend. You can make the choice for yourself and take the road less traveled and win the game of life! Everything will get better as you get stronger and more powerful and it all results from what fuel/food you put into your mouth. It really is that simple!*

When I arrived home from Mexico, I studied, and I found a few paths that I wanted to explore. The next part of this book will detail what I did and why, along with the amazing results.

Caveat: my experience is anecdotal in nature and represents only one man's journey back to health. In no way should you consider making any changes to your diet *unless you want to and unless it makes total sense to do so*. It might be wise to seek out a "functional doctor" before you embark on this journey to renewed health but ultimately, you are the one who is in control of your own health.

Chapter 6

The Day I Started on My Journey of Change

A few months had passed since I returned home with my vision. I'd finished my initial research and had the information I needed to formulate an approach that made sense to me. I was making a few lifestyle changes, like avoiding sweets and cutting back on alcohol, but I still hadn't jumped in with both feet. It was like getting into the ocean in California, which is cold. You first put your toe in and pull it back, then your foot and slowly you move forward until you're in the water swimming. It's a process. I was still working on my motivation and was still holding on to various aspects of my old life as I prepared my mind to accept what I was about to do. In other words, I was out on the edge of the 3-meter platform, looking down, contemplating making the leap, but still a little bit afraid, until one specific day when everything changed, and I took the leap. That day, I went to the movies. When I go to the movie theater, part of the experience for me had always been to eat my popcorn with a lot of butter. (Warning! This is disgusting!) When I say a lot of butter, this is what I mean. When I order the large bag, I make sure the people behind the counter know and understand that I am there for the butter, and by butter, I don't mean true natural butter from the farm. I mean the melted yellow lard-like substance that tastes a little like butter and goes great with salt and popcorn. I loved it! So, when I'd order my popcorn, I would invariably say something like this:

> *"I want a lot of butter with my popcorn, in fact, as far as I'm concerned, for me the popcorn is simply the delivery system for the butter. I want the butter pumped on in layers and if there isn't enough butter to penetrate the bottom of the bag and stain my pants, then I'm coming back to complain and get more butter!"*

I said this in jest, but I meant every word of it. Many times, I was forced to go back and get more butter. I was hooked on that "butter taste" experience.

On that day I followed my usual pattern and had a large bag of butter with some popcorn. An hour later, I definitely had my fill. Later that evening I went to dinner at my favorite Indian restaurant. I ordered my favorite dish, butter chicken. It's delicious but extremely hot, rich and spicy. But not to worry, I had taken my daily dose of Prilosec and I think, *I'm covered*. I was feeling fine when I went to bed, but at about 2am I woke up choking and coughing. I had to jump out of bed immediately and right my body. (Evidently, Prilosec has its limits and can only do so much.) I was experiencing a heartburn melt down. I've had this burning experience many times before and it's terrible. It always results from gluttony. Acid comes up from the stomach and into the esophagus where it burns and then it's immediately re-swallowed, burning again on its way back down. It's like fire burning in your throat. There is a reason why it's called heart*burn*. I went to the bathroom and tried to throw up. I couldn't stop coughing and spitting and every time I coughed, more acid would appear in my throat and burn. When I say *acid*, I'm talking hydrochloric acid! It can dissolve almost anything, pennies, nails . . . your esophagus.

(One of my earliest memories of my Father was of him pulling out his tums attempting to stop his chronic heartburn. He died young at 63 having contracted esophageal cancer.)

This cycle of acid coming up and burning and re-swallowing went on for over an hour or so before it calmed down enough for me to lay back down and go to sleep, but as soon as I laid down, it started coming up again. This ordeal went on for hours. I was mad as hell at myself for being so stupid and careless regarding what I put into my mouth that day. This episode was so disturbing that I made up my mind, once and for all, to begin the very next day on my detailed plan to change everything from the old eating habits and lifestyle to the new and enlightened healthy lifestyle plan I'd outlined for myself. When I got out of bed on the morning of March 7, 2018 (I'll never forget the day.) I was a new man. I had gone over to the edge, looked into the abyss and pulled back, changed by the experience. This was the beginning of my Journey in earnest.

It's unfortunate that it took such an ugly experience for me to be motivated enough to make serious changes to my diet. Some of us are stubborn and think we can game the system, but when it comes to the health of our bodies, it's just chemistry and chemistry is a science and it can't be fooled. I'm thankful now for that experience that took me to the end of my rope, and I'm hoping that you are smarter than I was and it won't be necessary for you to reach such a point of gluttony that is so ugly and painful that the experience changes your perception forever . . . but, whatever it takes to make the change, I promise you, it will always be worth it!

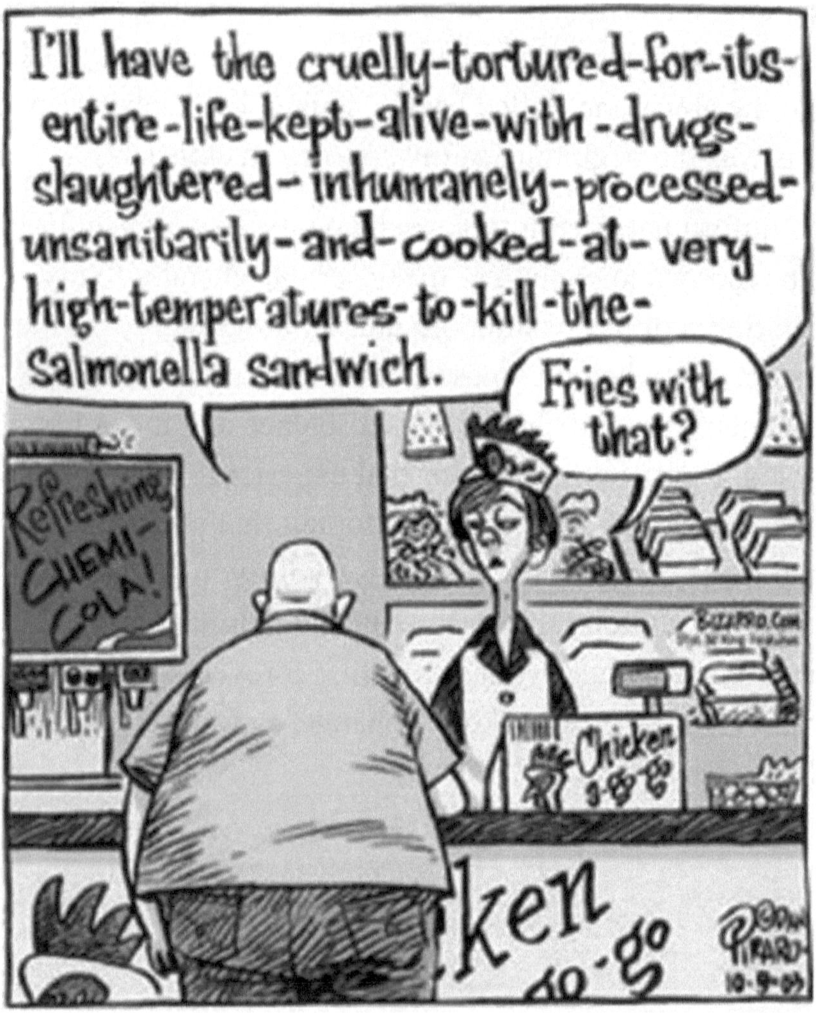

I'll have the cruelly-tortured-for-its-entire-life-kept-alive-with-drugs-slaughtered-inhumanely-processed-unsanitarily-and-cooked-at-very-high-temperatures-to-kill-the-salmonella sandwich.
Fries with that?
Refreshing CHEMI-COLA!
Chicken 3-&-Go
ken to-go

Chapter 7

The Healing Begins!

The Leaky Gut!

Now I knew what I needed to do, and I was willing to do it. I started with my so called "leaky gut." There has been a lot of talk about this subject recently. You can't find it in a medical text book and some traditional doctors still doubt its existence, but the science behind the leaky gut is becoming clearer and more medical professionals are jumping on board this current bandwagon. One of my personal *functional doctors*, Dr. Adam Fields, is a specialist in the area of fixing one's gut. The basic concept is this:

A lot of health problems, especially autoimmune diseases, are caused by having a leaky gut so it's imperative to start here. You don't keep pouring water into a leaky bucket. First, you fix the hole, and then you put water in it. A possible cause of leaky gut is increased intestinal permeability or intestinal hyperpermeability. That could happen when tight junctions in the gut, which control what passes through the lining of the small intestine, don't work properly. That could let *toxic* substances leak into the bloodstream. These substances, pieces of undigested food and large chain protein molecules are then seen as "foreign invaders" by our immune system and are attacked by our white blood cells. This causes inflammation that may lead to autoimmune diseases.

If you remember, I had an autoimmune disease called Polymyalgia Rheumatica or PMR. As I said, many "functional" doctors see a direct connection between having a leaky gut and autoimmune diseases.* (*The Autoimmune Epidemic* by Dr. Donna Nakazawa, MD) So this seemed like a good place to start.

Based on my research and the advice of my functional doctor, I chose to start with my gut and find a way to heal it. Here is some amazing new science through which they have discovered that the gut holds a high and lofty place of importance in our bodies. That discovery makes the case for getting your gut right. This is of primary importance.

The gut to brain connection is no joke; anxiety has been linked to stomach problems *and* the stomach has been linked to anxiety issues. Have you ever had a "gut-wrenching" experience? Do certain situations make you "feel nauseous"? Have you ever felt "butterflies" in your stomach? We use these expressions for a reason. The gastrointestinal tract is sensitive to emotion. Anger, anxiety, sadness, elation, all of these feelings (and others) can trigger symptoms in the gut.

The brain has a direct effect on the stomach and intestines. For example, the very thought of eating can release the stomach's juices before food gets there. This connection goes both ways. A troubled intestine can send signals to the brain, just as a troubled brain can send signals to the gut. Therefore, a person's stomach or intestinal distress can be the cause *or* the product of anxiety, stress, or depression. That's because the brain and the gastrointestinal (GI) system are intimately connected. So, when you are healing your gut, you are helping your brain to work more efficiently as well . . . and we all want that, right?

I was committed, but first, one of my other functional doctors, Jay Pennock M.D., wanted me to do a "poop test". This is gross but necessary. You have this bio-hazard kit with 5 pairs of latex gloves and small carboard boxes to collect your poop over a 5-day period. This is very scientific. The kit came with directions but there is no learning curve here. You better get it right the first time or . . . well you get the idea. The reason for the test is so that we can see what kinds of bacteria are currently living in your intestines. This way, you can evaluate the current condition of the gut's "garden" to see the kinds and concentrations of bacteria that are residing there and which new ones you'll need to add to your gut flora, or gastrointestinal *microbiota* which is the complex community of microorganisms that live in the digestive tracts of humans and other animals, including insects.

Wikipedia defines microbiota as an:

> "... ecological community of
> commensal, symbiotic and
> pathogenic microorganisms
> found in and on all multicellular
> organisms studied to date from
> plants to animals. A microbiota
> includes bacteria, archaea,
> protists, fungi and viruses."

The composition of the human gut microbiota changes over time, when the diet changes, and as overall health changes. Dr. Jay Pennock, MD, my other "functional" doctor told me that, with this test kit, we would establish a base line from which to build. It turned out I had a lot of bad bacteria, but no parasites, which is good. Unfortunately, the bacteria I had were the kind that like to eat McDonalds hamburgers and French fries — not the best kind. We needed to overwhelm the bad guys with the new good ones I'd be adding to my gut flora. Here is the basic protocol to heal a leaky gut:

> The first thing to do is start taking a good probiotic. The easiest way to get the proper probiotics is to take it in capsules that contain billions and billions of micro-organisms that are the good bacteria that become the gate keepers of our gut. (There are many ways to get probiotics into your gut, but the capsules

are easy and pack a lot of beneficial bacteria into a small space.) When one takes a proper dose over a period of time, it's like bringing in reinforcements to the area that needs help. Think about it this way, when you add the probiotics to your diet, the good guys are coming over the hill to save the day. They will destroy the bad bacteria and create a new and healthy nutrient-loving garden in your intestines. And, they will close off the weak areas in your gut and prevent substances from leaking out of the gut and into the blood stream.

This was the first step I tried in conjunction with changing my diet. I learned what foods would be good and protective and healing to my gut and what foods were destructive to my gut. Here is a partial list:

Great Food Options for Fixing a Leaky Gut

- **Vegetables:** Broccoli, Brussels sprouts, cabbage, arugula, carrots, kale, eggplant, beetroot, Swiss chard, spinach, ginger, mushrooms and zucchini.
- **Roots and tubers:** Potatoes, sweet potatoes, yams, carrots, squash and turnips.
- **Fermented vegetables:** Kimchi, sauerkraut, tempeh and miso.

- **Fruit:** Coconut, grapes, bananas, blueberries, raspberries, strawberries, kiwi, pineapple, oranges, mandarin, lemon, limes, passionfruit and papaya.
- **Sprouted seeds:** Chia seeds, flax seeds, sunflower seeds and more.
- **Gluten-free grains:** Buckwheat, amaranth, rice (brown and white), sorghum, and gluten-free oats.
- **Healthy fats:** Avocado, avocado oil, coconut oil and extra virgin olive oil.
- **Fish:** Salmon, tuna, herring and other omega-3-rich fish.
- **Herbs and spices:** All herbs and spices.
- **Cultured dairy products:** Kefir, yogurt, Greek yogurt and traditional buttermilk – (some people don't like to take any milk products at all. I didn't for the first two months and added some yogurt in after that with no problems.)
- **Beverages:** Bone broth, teas, coconut milk, nut milk, water and kombucha.
- **Nuts:** Raw nuts including peanuts, almonds and nut-based products, such as nut milks.

Some Foods to Avoid

The following list contains foods that *may harm healthy gut bacteria,* as well as some that are believed to *trigger digestive symptoms, such as bloating, constipation and diarrhea:*

- **Wheat-based products:** Bread, pasta, cereals, wheat flour, couscous, etc.
- **Gluten-containing grains:** Barley, rye, bulgur, seitan, triticale and oats.
- **Processed meats:** Cold cuts, deli meats, bacon, hot dogs, etc.
- **Red Meat**
- **Baked goods:** Cakes, muffins, cookies, pies, pastries and pizza.
- **Snack foods:** Crackers, muesli bars, popcorn, pretzels, etc.
- **Junk food:** Fast foods, potato chips, sugary cereals, candy bars, etc.
- **Dairy products:** Milk, cheeses and ice cream.
- **Refined oils:** Canola, sunflower, soybean and safflower oils.
- **Artificial sweeteners:** Aspartame, sucralose and saccharin.
- **Sauces:** Salad dressings, as well as soy, teriyaki and hoisin sauce.
- **Beverages:** Alcohol, carbonated beverages and other sugary drinks.

It's so simple: eat healthy, mostly plant-based food and don't eat unhealthy *food-like* substances. No fast food or processed food. Simple, right?

OK, I know it's not so simple. Over the years, our bodies have built up strong cravings for certain foods that aren't building you up but are in fact tearing you down. We know this, but we order the deep-fried French fries anyway because we crave them. So it looks simple on paper, but it's not going to be easy. This is where the rubber meets the road. *Oh no!* you say, *Not the diet part!* Yes, *the diet part* but think "lifestyle" and not diet. It's a way of life and a way of thinking about food that counts. Knowing the truth about food and what it's for and how it works with your system, will take you a long way toward a successful transition to optimum health. Education, learning, and knowledge will lead you to the truth and knowing the truth will facilitate the needed lifestyle change.

What goes into your mouth should be of utmost importance to you because it goes into your stomach and gut, is fully processed and feeds your body. That specific food you put into your mouth obviously makes an impact on your body and how you feel and ultimately on your overall health. Why not give your body its best chance for a long and healthy life? It's a simple understanding, but somehow there is often a disconnect between what we know is good for us and what we actually do. We need to overcome that disconnect and the way to do that is to become educated. Again, *the truth will set you free!*

Chapter 8

The Lifestyle "Diet"

After much research, I came to the simple conclusion that a lifestyle change would go a long way toward healthy living. After all the diets and modalities and health paths to choose from, I decided on the basic whole-food, plant-based diet and lifestyle. What's that? Just what it sounds like. It turns out that the foods you need to eat and need to avoid, that are listed above to repair and promote a healthy gut, are very similar to what you'll find when eating a whole-food, plant-based diet. Again, it's simple — eat food that grows out of the soil and avoid processed foods completely. Cakes, cookies, pies, pasta, bread and anything else that comes in a box from the supermarket, is processed and, therefore, is off the list.

Keep in mind, I was seeking out a diet with the purpose of getting well, restoring myself to optimum health, becoming disease free and ultimately free of all prescription medications and their endless side-effects. If you are being motivated to make healthy lifestyle changes to heal or reverse a specific disease, in the beginning it's important to be as compliant as possible, sticking to the plan and eating clean. Based on my extensive research, I believe that most chronic diseases such as type 2 diabetes, most autoimmune diseases, heart disease, and many cancers can be reversed or eliminated altogether by following a plant-based diet, and here is the great part, you can be healed in a matter of weeks, 6 to 10 weeks for most health issues, even of type 2 diabetes! So, you don't necessarily have to be on this new strange, seemingly restrictive lifestyle diet for years before you see its results. Every human body loves what you'll be feeding yours and its response will be quick and amazing. Your new choice in food will seem somewhat radical in today's world, but it's actually the most natural way to eat. After you are healed and well (and as I said, you can be well in only 6 to 10 weeks with this lifestyle change) you can slowly bring back into your diet foods that do not necessarily promote optimum health but if eaten sparingly, our bodies will successfully process the "poisons" and you'll recover without too much damage. It's up to you but be sensitive to how your body reacts. Be aware of how you are feeling, especially after you eat.

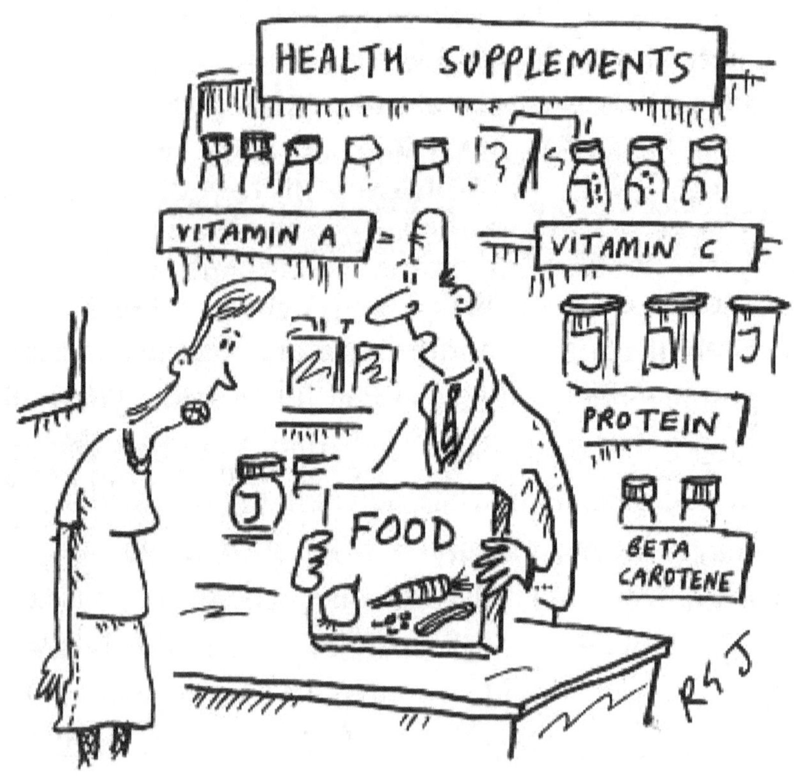

"Have you tried this? It used to be all the rage"

If anything you eat gives you brain fog or makes you sluggish, notice that and make the appropriate changes. Once you get healthy, you will have a new view of what food is and you'll be making wise decisions based on your new knowledge and understanding of what works best for you.

Simply put, during the first 6 to 8 weeks, stick firmly to the plan of eating fruits and veggies mostly and avoid all processed foods, breads, red meat, sugar of all kinds (except fruit), dairy products and alcohol. If it comes in a box, don't eat it.

Again, it's not going to be easy. For most people, changing their diet to a plant-based lifestyle is hard to imagine. It certainly was for me. I loved my red meat, I loved my sweets, I loved my pasta . . . but green leafy vegetables - not so much. In fact, twenty-five years ago, my health-conscious cousin Adam gave me John Robins' book *Diet for a New America*. I put it aside unread when I realized it was about the horrors of eating meat. I saw where the book was going, and I didn't want to go there. I stopped reading because I didn't want to change, and I didn't even want to know the truth about the meat industry or anything that would lessen my desire or inclination to eat meat. I loved red meat and steaks of all kinds. (When I barbecued a steak, half of it was eaten before I brought it to the table. I just couldn't wait.) So, I lived and ate in willful ignorance and was happy for a time, most of my life in fact. Unfortunately, for me, it took getting sick to get my attention. I'm hoping some of you reading this book, who are not sick, will be wiser than I was. But here is the good news! Once I made the decision to stop eating red meat, it wasn't really that hard. It's all about making the decision and knowing why you are doing such a thing, and all of a

sudden . . . meat's off the plate and not really missed.
Honest to goodness. I don't think about it anymore.

You Have Complete Control!

Philosophical Comment

You are in control of this one thing in life: *You get to choose what goes in your mouth.*

Life can be difficult and hard to navigate at times. Figuring out one's goals in life — who to marry, what job to pursue, where to live — these are all big decisions common to most of us and these life decisions have a lot of variables and outside factors of influence - voices and opinions that can impact your decision-making one way or another. In other words, you do not have as much control over your life as you think you do, but when it comes to your health, it's all up to you! The emphasis is on you. You are in total control of what you put into your mouth every time, every day. The point is, you are the only one who has this control, and no one can really change that fact or keep you from becoming healthy if you choose to go there. Do you want to be a more powerful person in every way? Practice being a powerful person by making smart choices for your health and that power will overflow into the rest of your life. Those wise choices will lead you to make other wise choices and before you know it, you'll be a more powerful person in every area of your life.

OK, it all sounds good but still, for some reason it's not easy to do. Why? Because most people lack the knowledge and understanding necessary to move them toward making the wise daily decisions that are in their own best interest. It starts and ends with knowledge and education, which, hopefully, is why you are reading this book. The more knowledge you have, the easier it will be to make the right decisions. It takes practice. Few of us can change overnight, but you'll get a lot of chances to get it right, three times a day . . . every day!

And even when we begin to understand the importance and value of clean and right eating, it still takes a major effort to make the changes. Why? Are we just weak human beings? Yes, but we can become stronger and wiser concerning our health. For me it started with knowledge and understanding of the simple basics like: *What is food really for*? Start with getting educated and being open to the possibility of being a more powerful human being. We know we are what we eat, or actually, what we absorb in our gut, but we are also what we *eat* or take in mentally, what we are listening to, what we are reading and who are we talking to and associating with. You need to feed your mind with truth and positive information in order to change it. We need to overcome the old patterns of behavior with new ideas and truth that will lead us to a better place. It helps a lot if we know what we are doing and why. I can help you with this, but ultimately, it's up to you. The goal in life is to be better human beings. We are given a lifetime to make improvements and that's part of why we are here. To think and grow and be a hero if possible. It could happen, you never know until you try and that's the point. Isn't one of life's primary goals to try to be a better, stronger, more powerful and happier loving human being? Of course, it is! It's what life is all about. Keep that in mind at all times and this lifestyle change will help in all of these areas and . . . it's totally worth the effort. That is my promise. By its healing nature, your lifestyle change will create "new streams in the desert" and expand your experience of life and enhance your personal reality . . . and that's a good thing!

Back to my healing story. The first step for me was taking the probiotics and that was easy. It helps to get the right probiotics, I got mine from my holistic functional doctor, Dr. Adam Fields of "Fields Family Chiropractic". He recommended Microbiome, a leader in pharmaceutical grade products. I took an assortment of probiotics over an 8-week period. Again, the purpose of this action was to repopulate my gut with the beneficial bacteria known for enhancing good digestion and healing the gut. I was repairing the holes in the small intestine where partially digested food particles were leaking into the bloodstream causing an inflammatory immune response and my autoimmune disease. Once I started the probiotics, I focused on what else I put into my mouth. I took the probiotics to heal the gut and ate healing foods that were soothing and didn't exacerbate the problem. **<u>Healing foods combined with healing bacteria was step one.</u>**

Chapter 9

Weight Loss!

About Being Satisfied and Losing Weight

It's a fact that when you are eating foods loaded with nutrients you become satisfied easily and you just aren't that hungry. You eat when hungry and not out of habit or because "it's time". For me, after a week on the plant-based diet, I noticed I wasn't that hungry, and I didn't eat that much when I did eat. As a result I noticed that I was losing weight. Almost a pound a day! When I started this diet, I

was 170 lbs. and at 5'8," I was over my ideal weight and had a good beer belly going. By the end of the initial six weeks of being on a good healthy plant-based diet, I had lost 15 lbs. and was down to 155 lbs. This was amazing because I hadn't been that thin for over 25 years! My body went back to its normal weight for my height and bone structure and I even looked decent in my t-shirts again. Not a bad side effect to the plant-based diet. Losing weight was not a goal when I approached this new lifestyle, it just happened. I eventually went to a low of 149 lbs. but bounced back to a new normal range of between 151 and 155 pounds. I've maintained this ideal weight over the past year without even thinking about it.

The 5-2 Diet

As I was researching ways to get healthy, I came across what is called the 5-2 diet. I was attracted to it because of its simplicity. Here is how it works. You eat whatever you want for any 5 days of the week and do a full or partial fast for two days. This was appealing to me because you only need to be disciplined for a couple of days and the other 5 days of the week you just eat a normal diet (hopefully reasonably healthy). The **5-2 diet**, also known as The Fast Diet, is currently the most popular intermittent fasting diet. It was popularized by British journalist Michael Mosley. It's called the 5:2 diet because five days of the week are normal eating days, while the other two restrict calories to 500–600 per day. Restricting calories for two days weekly works well for many people because it gives the digestive system a chance to rest, repair and expel excess. Your body regenerates and increases its metabolism when you cut calories, whereas when you completely cut food it goes into starvation mode, storing fat and slowing metabolism. Intermittent calorie restriction also allows your elastic stomach to return to its normal size, so you tend not to overindulge. You can learn more about this by searching out the "5-2 diet" on YouTube. I mention this diet because for some, it may be an easier approach to getting healthy and ultimately, loosing excess weight is a good start on the road back to health, but it is more of a "diet" vs. a lifestyle and I believe it's better to live a healthy lifestyle than to be on a "diet".

Fasting?

A little more on the idea of fasting. The idea behind fasting is easy to understand. When you go for a prolonged period of time between meals you give your body/digestive system a much-needed rest. While resting, your stomach and all your individual cells get the chance to heal. This process promotes health and vitality in your cells and your body. I did some fasting while on my strict 8-week diet, but I did it simply because I wasn't hungry and skipped meals, sometimes two meals in a row, taking me to the 16 to 18 hours of partial fasting that some say will create a healing and resting period for your cells. I didn't follow the 5-2 diet in any organized way. I mention it here just to let you know I was aware of the fact that, in the first few months, I was doing partial fasts without planning for them. It just came about because I simply wasn't that hungry, and I didn't eat unless I was hungry, therefore I lost weight. Here is a secret: when you eliminate sugar from your diet, you aren't that hungry anymore. Sugar causes over eating and cravings for more sugar and almost everything in the Standard American Diet (the SAD diet) has sugar in it. After only a week of being off sugar, the cravings go away and that makes life so much easier. The pull of sugar is powerful, but it can be defeated by the will: "Just say no!" You can learn and change your habits. It gets easier each day until you don't think about it anymore. If I can do it, anyone can. The best news is that the body is amazing when it has the right fuel. With the right diet and lifestyle changes, your body will quickly reset/reboot itself. Try it and see for yourself. You won't be sorry, and you *will* be astounded.

Because sugar is such a big part of our modern diet and responsible for so much sickness and disease, we're going to take a deep dive into the subject. Remember, learning, knowledge and understanding is going to be the secret to your success in this undertaking. Get ready, you are going to become an expert on sugar and know why you don't want to include it in your new lifestyle.

Chapter 10

Sugar = Poison

At this point in my journey back to health, I was taking a full regimen of high-grade probiotics and I began to change my daily eating habits like cutting out all sugar from my diet. If you currently have a sweet tooth, there is no way to "sugar coat" this, but sugar is very bad for you and could actually be the worst component of your current diet. Some put it up there on the same level as poison and call it the "white plague" or the "white death". The side effects of eating a lot of sugar are too many to list here, but just google "sugar is poison" and start reading. I know, saying, "No," to sugar isn't easy so I've listed below some scientific reasons why you should avoid eating excess sugar. Convince your mind over and over with evidence, knowledge and logic and you are halfway there.

11 Reasons Why Too Much Sugar Is Bad for You

From marinara sauce to peanut butter, added sugar can be found in even the most unexpected products. Many people rely on quick, processed foods for meals and snacks. Since these products often contain added sugar, it makes up a large proportion of their daily calorie intake. In the US, added sugars account for up to 17% of the total calorie intake of adults and up to 14% for children. Dietary guidelines suggest limiting calories from added sugar to less than 10% per day. Experts believe that sugar consumption is a major cause of obesity and many chronic diseases, such as diabetes. Here are 11 reasons why eating too much sugar is bad for your health:

1. Can Cause Weight Gain

Rates of obesity are rising worldwide and added sugar, especially from sugar-sweetened beverages, is thought to be one of the main culprits. Sugar-sweetened drinks like sodas, juices and sweet teas are loaded with fructose, a type of simple sugar. Consuming fructose increases your hunger and desire for food more than glucose, the main type of sugar found in starchy foods. Additionally, excessive fructose consumption may cause resistance to leptin, an important hormone that regulates hunger and tells your body to stop eating. In other words, sugary beverages don't curb your hunger, making it easy to quickly consume a high number of liquid calories. This can lead to weight gain. Research has consistently shown that people who drink sugary beverages, such as soda and juice, weigh more than people who don't. Also, drinking a lot of sugar-sweetened beverages is linked to an increased amount of visceral fat, a kind of deep belly fat associated with conditions like diabetes and heart disease.

SUMMARY: Consuming too much added sugar, especially from sugary beverages, increases your risk of weight gain and can lead to visceral fat accumulation.

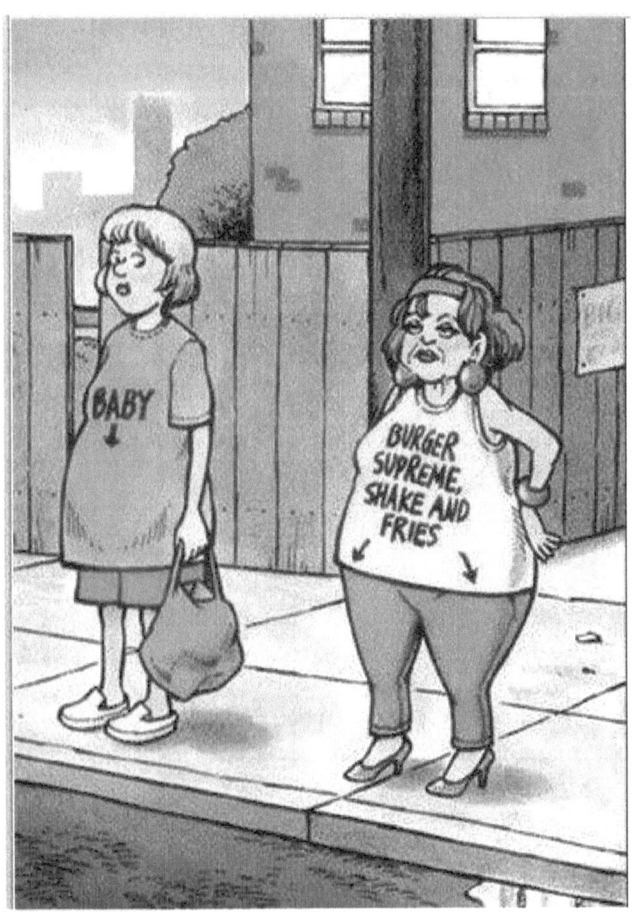

2. May Increase Your Risk of Heart Disease

High-sugar diets have been associated with an increased risk of many diseases, including heart disease, the number one cause of death worldwide. Evidence suggests that high-sugar diets can lead to obesity, inflammation and high levels of triglycerides, high blood sugar and high blood pressure, which are all risk factors for heart disease. Additionally, consuming too much sugar, especially from sugar-sweetened drinks, has been linked to atherosclerosis, a disease characterized by fatty, artery-clogging deposits. A study in over 30,000 people found that those who consumed 17–21% of calories from added sugar had a 38% greater risk of dying from heart disease, compared to those consuming only 8% of calories from added sugar. Just one 16-ounce (473-ml) can of soda contains 52 grams of sugar, which equates to more than 10% of your daily calorie consumption, based on a 2,000-calorie diet. This means that one sugary drink a day can already put you over the recommended daily limit for added sugar.

SUMMARY: Consuming too much added sugar increases heart disease risk factors such as obesity, high blood pressure and inflammation. High-sugar diets have been linked to an increased risk of dying from heart disease.

3. Has Been Linked to Acne

A diet high in refined carbs, including sugary foods and drinks, has been associated with a higher risk of developing acne. Foods with a high glycemic index, such as processed sweets, raise your blood sugar more rapidly than foods with a lower glycemic index. Sugary foods quickly spike blood sugar and insulin levels, causing increased androgen secretion, oil production and inflammation, all of which play a role in acne development. Studies have shown that low-glycemic diets are associated with a reduced acne risk, while high-glycemic diets are linked to a greater risk. For example, a study in 2,300 teens demonstrated that those who frequently consumed added sugar had a 30% greater risk of developing acne.

Also, many population studies have shown that rural communities that consume traditional, non-processed foods have almost non-existent rates of acne, compared to more urban, high-income areas. These findings coincide with the theory that diets high in processed, sugar-laden foods contribute to the development of acne.

SUMMARY: High-sugar diets can increase androgen secretion, oil production and inflammation, all of which can raise your risk of developing acne.

4. Increases Your Risk of Diabetes

The worldwide prevalence of diabetes has more than doubled over the past 30 years. Though there are many reasons for this, there is a clear link between excessive sugar consumption and diabetes risk. Obesity, which is often caused by consuming too much sugar, is considered the strongest risk factor for diabetes. What's more, prolonged high-sugar consumption drives resistance to insulin, a hormone produced by the pancreas that regulates blood sugar levels. Insulin resistance causes blood sugar levels to rise and strongly increases your risk of diabetes. A population study comprising over 175 countries found that the risk of developing diabetes grew by 1.1% for every 150 calories of sugar, or about one can of soda, consumed per day. Other studies have also shown that people who drink sugar-sweetened beverages, including fruit juice, are more likely to develop diabetes.

SUMMARY: A high-sugar diet may lead to obesity and insulin resistance, both of which are risk factors for diabetes.

5. May Increase Your Risk of Cancer

Eating excessive amounts of sugar may increase your risk of developing certain cancers. First, a diet laden with sugary foods and beverages can lead to obesity, which significantly raises your risk of cancer. Furthermore, diets high in sugar increase inflammation in your body and may cause insulin resistance, both of which increase cancer risk. A study in over 430,000 people found that added sugar consumption was positively associated with an increased risk of esophageal cancer, pleural cancer and cancer of the small intestine. Another study showed that women who consumed sweet buns and cookies more than three times per week were 1.42 times more likely to develop endometrial cancer than women who consumed these foods less than 0.5 times per week. Research on the link between added sugar intake and cancer is ongoing, and more studies are needed to fully understand this complex relationship.

SUMMARY: Too much sugar can lead to obesity, insulin resistance and inflammation, all of which are known to be risk factors for cancer.

6. *May Increase Your Risk of Depression*

While a healthy diet can help improve your mood, a diet high in added sugar and processed foods may increase your chances of developing depression. Consuming a lot of processed foods, including high-sugar products such as cakes and sugary drinks, has been associated with a higher risk of depression. Researchers believe that blood sugar swings, neurotransmitter dysregulation and inflammation may all be reasons for sugar's detrimental impact on mental health. A study following 8,000 people for 22 years showed that men who consumed 67 grams or more of sugar per day were 23% more likely to develop depression than men who ate less than 40 grams per day. Another study in over 69,000 women demonstrated that those with the highest intakes of added sugars had a significantly greater risk of depression, compared to those with the lowest intakes.

SUMMARY: A diet rich in added sugar and processed foods may increase depression risk in both men and women.

7. May Accelerate the Skin Aging Process

Wrinkles are a natural sign of aging. They appear eventually, regardless of your health. However, poor food choices can worsen wrinkles and speed the skin's aging process. Advanced glycation end products (AGEs) are compounds formed by reactions between sugar and protein in your body. They are suspected to play a key role in skin aging. Consuming a diet high in refined carbs and sugar leads to the production of AGEs, which may cause your skin to age prematurely. AGEs damage collagen and elastin, which are proteins that help the skin stretch and keep its youthful appearance. When collagen and elastin become damaged, the skin loses its firmness and begins to sag. In one study, women who consumed more carbs, including added sugars, had a more wrinkled appearance than women on a high-protein, lower-carb diet. The researchers concluded that a lower intake of carbs was associated with better skin-aging appearance.

SUMMARY: Sugary foods can increase the production of AGEs, which can accelerate skin aging and wrinkle formation.

8. Can Increase Cellular Aging

Telomeres are structures found at the end of chromosomes, which are molecules that hold part or all of your genetic information. Telomeres act as protective caps, preventing chromosomes from deteriorating or fusing together. As you grow older, telomeres naturally shorten, which causes cells to age and malfunction. Although the shortening of telomeres is a normal part of aging, unhealthy lifestyle choices can speed up the process. Consuming high amounts of sugar has been shown to accelerate telomere shortening, which increases cellular aging. A study in 5,309 adults showed that regularly drinking sugar-sweetened beverages was associated with shorter telomere length and premature cellular aging. In fact, each daily 20-ounce (591-ml) serving of sugar-sweetened soda equated to 4.6 additional years of aging, independent of other variables.

SUMMARY: Eating too much sugar can accelerate the shortening of telomeres, which increases cellular aging.

9. Drains Your Energy

Foods high in added sugar quickly spike blood sugar and insulin levels, leading to increased energy in the short term. However, this rise in energy levels is fleeting. Products that are loaded with sugar but lacking in protein, fiber or fat lead to a brief energy boost that's quickly followed by a sharp drop in blood sugar, often referred to as a crash. Having constant blood sugar swings can lead to major fluctuations in energy levels. To avoid this energy-draining cycle, choose carb sources that are low in added sugar and rich in fiber. Pairing carbs with protein or fat is another great way to keep your blood sugar and energy levels stable. For example, eating an apple along with a small handful of almonds is an excellent snack for prolonged, consistent energy levels.

SUMMARY: High-sugar foods can negatively impact your energy levels by causing a spike in blood sugar followed quickly by a crash.

10. Can Lead to Fatty Liver

A high intake of fructose has been consistently linked to an increased risk of fatty liver. Unlike glucose and other types of sugar, which are taken up by many cells throughout the body, fructose is almost exclusively broken down by the liver. In the liver, fructose is converted into energy or stored as glycogen. However, the liver can only store so much glycogen before excess amounts are turned into fat. Large amounts of added sugar in the form of fructose overload your liver, leading to non-alcoholic fatty liver disease (NAFLD), a condition characterized by excessive fat buildup in the liver. A study in over 5,900 adults showed that people who drank sugar-sweetened beverages daily had a 56% higher risk of developing NAFLD, compared to people who did not.

SUMMARY: Eating too much sugar may lead to NAFLD, a condition in which excessive fat builds up in the liver.

11. Other Health Risks

Aside from the risks listed above, sugar can harm your body in countless other ways. Research shows that too much added sugar can:

- **Increase kidney disease risk:** Having consistently high blood sugar levels can cause damage to the delicate blood vessels in your kidneys. This can lead to an increased risk of kidney disease.
- **Negatively impact dental health:** Eating too much sugar can cause cavities. Bacteria in your mouth feed on sugar and release acid byproducts, which cause tooth demineralization.
- **Increase the risk of developing gout:** Gout is an inflammatory condition characterized by pain in the

joints. Added sugars raise uric acid levels in the blood, increasing the risk of developing or worsening gout.

- **Accelerate cognitive decline:** High-sugar diets can lead to impaired memory and have been linked to an increased risk of dementia.

Research on the impact of added sugar on health is ongoing, and new discoveries are constantly being made.

SUMMARY: Consuming too much sugar may worsen cognitive decline, increase gout risk, harm your kidneys and cause cavities.

I kept thinking "one thing leads to another", i.e. sugar to insulin. Insulin to obesity. Obesity to inflammation. Inflammation to diabetes and then to cancer!

So, now we know that sugar is something to be avoided, right? Let's look at a few ways to do this.

How to Reduce Your Sugar Intake

OK, if we didn't know already . . . we certainly know now . . . excessive added sugar has many negative health effects. Although consuming small amounts now and then is perfectly fine because your body can handle it in small quantities over time, you should try to cut back on sugar whenever possible. Fortunately, simply focusing on eating whole, unprocessed foods automatically decreases the amount of sugar in your diet. Here are some tips on how to reduce your intake of added sugars:

- Swap sodas, energy drinks, juices and sweetened teas for water or unsweetened seltzer, heated bone broth, Kombucha.
- Drink your coffee black or use Stevia for a zero-calorie, natural sweetener.
- Sweeten plain yogurt with fresh or frozen berries instead of buying flavored, sugar-loaded yogurt.
- Consume whole fruits instead of sugar-sweetened fruit smoothies.
- Replace candy with a homemade trail mix of fruit, nuts and a few dark chocolate chips.
- Use olive oil and vinegar in place of sweet salad dressings like honey mustard.
- Choose marinades, nut butters, ketchup and marinara sauce with zero added sugars.
- Look for cereals, granolas and granola bars with under 4 grams of sugar per serving.
- Swap your morning cereal for a bowl of rolled oats topped with nut butter and fresh berries, or an omelet made with fresh greens.
- Instead of jelly, slice fresh bananas onto your peanut butter sandwich.
- Use natural nut butters in place of sweet spreads like Nutella.
- Avoid alcoholic beverages that are sweetened with soda, juice, honey, sugar or agave.

- Shop the perimeter of the grocery store, focusing on fresh, whole ingredients.

As I mentioned before, keeping a food diary is an excellent way of becoming more aware of the main sources of sugar in your diet. The best way to limit your added sugar intake is to prepare your own healthy meals at home and avoid buying foods and drinks that are high in added sugar. In fact, I found it helpful to never buy any food product that is not on my "healthy" list and that way I'm not tempted to eat something that is off limits. If it's off limits, it's not in the house. Out of sight out of mind actually works.

SUMMARY: Focusing on preparing healthy meals and limiting your intake of foods that contain added sweeteners can help you cut back on the amount of sugar in your diet and cut back on your out-of-control appetite.

The Bottom Line

Eating too much added sugar can have many negative health effects. If you haven't guessed yet, *sugar is the single worst "food" you have in your diet, period!* We all know that changing anything that is habitual is hard, very hard, but making the difficult changes is necessary if you want to be your best self. And please know, I personally and deeply understand that making changes like cutting sugar and red meat out of your diet isn't easy and in fact this is the part I avoided all my life and is probably why I got sick in the first place! I kept thinking "one thing leads to another", i.e. sugar to insulin. Insulin to obesity. Obesity to inflammation. Inflammation to diabetes and autoimmune diseases then to cancer. Ouch!

]

Chapter 11

The Question of Meat

This is a tough one! The very idea of not eating red meat made me turn away from any attempt to change to a plant-based diet. It's hard for me to imagine that anyone could love eating meat more than me. So, this was my biggest hurdle. How did I do it? When you get to the place where being healthy and vital is of higher value than eating meat, you'll have little problem moving on to greener pastures. Investigate for yourself and find the truth behind what you are eating and keep that thought in mind. I removed meat from my diet because after the extensive reading and knowledge I acquired while on my quest, I knew if I wanted to get my health back, I needed to give up meat, at least for the time being. For the first 8 weeks of my new diet and lifestyle the only meat I ate was wild salmon, which I enjoyed when out with friends at a restaurant or occasionally at home. Wild salmon seems benign in its negative effects compared to red meat and it's more sustainable as a food source compared to beef. It's also loaded with beneficial oils, Omega 3's and essential fatty acids. There are many Vegans who don't eat meat strictly because they don't believe in killing animals to feed themselves, others are into the poor performance in the sustainability aspect of beef. This refers to the idea that it takes too many resources in water, grass, feed and space, and that's why they choose not to eat beef or meat of any kind.

For me, I removed beef from my plate because I want to be healthy and eating beef comes with a host of negative inputs for the body and its systems.

There is no doubt that eating meat creates health concerns not only for consumers but also for the environment and (of course) the farmed animals, and it's unfortunate that people overlook so many of these problems. Animals are taken advantage of, the environment suffers, and ultimately you suffer, as well.

An animal-based diet isn't as diverse in terms of nutrients as a plant-based diet is. You pretty much get two main macronutrients — protein and fat — with essentially no vitamins or minerals, and no fiber. What most people don't know is that the body needs vitamins and minerals to digest and assimilate protein efficiently. Bodies also need fiber to help push things through and assimilate nutrients.

Meat intake can build up in the body and slow things down, causing you to feel tired and undernourished. Going plant-based ensures that your body at least gets the nutritional baseline it requires to thrive on a day-to-day basis. Meat is one of the major acidic foods in the standard North American diet. It's difficult for the body to break down and digest and requires extra work from the kidneys. As a result, it produces too much acid in the body. Too much acid not only weakens the body's immune defenses, which increases risks for infections, but also contributes to chronic diseases.

The other consideration to look at is the *quality* of meat that a majority of people eat: often it's fried, overcooked, and not eaten alongside green vegetables. This not only creates acidity in the body but also does nothing to help neutralize it. Choosing to eat more plants throughout the day can help balance this ratio.

So, the list goes on and on. If you are into getting really healthy, eating a lot of red meat will not get you there and in fact can hold you back from your best self.

This is not to say that I will never eat red meat again but if I do it will not be a primary aspect of my diet but rather a rare "treat" eaten under special circumstances. The main focus should be on the "lifestyle" of eating mostly a plant-based diet and avoiding foods that do little to keep you healthy and fit. So, having an occasional food that is not plant based may be OK if you don't make a habit of it. For example, Casey, my son-in-law lives in the Pacific Northwest and is an avid hunter. If I'm visiting and he's barbecuing deer steaks, I'm going to have one. Fresh

Venison has no anti-biotics or chemicals injected into them. They are purely "grass feed" and it's my belief that eating meat very occasionally will have a mostly benign affect on the human body. This leads into my next concern.

Relax! Don't be a Food Nazi:

I want to be completely honest here. Many "purists" may not agree with this. It has to do with being invited to friends' homes for dinner. I made the decision that when invited over to a friend's home for dinner, I would eat whatever was served to me, regardless of the dish. If it was meat, I ate it and thanked my hosts and appreciated the rare change in my diet and was actually happy to have the opportunity to eat some forbidden food. This included eating dessert. I ate it and appreciated it and was thankful for it! I think of this as a chance to "let off some steam" so to speak regarding my overall eating habits. This attitude came about after my first 8 weeks of strict eating and after my gut-healing time. But after being healed, I became less regimented when eating out. My reasoning was that I didn't want to "food-shame" people. As it was, when my friends saw me reject a certain food, they apologized and began to make excuses for their own eating habits . . . and I didn't like making people feel uncomfortable. I know lifestyle changes happen when people are ready to make the changes, and not until then. When I share my healing story, it's with the idea that some percentage of the people who hear the story will be ready and interested and want to learn what they can to be uber healthy themselves. It's those people I'm reaching out to. As I'm writing this, I'm still only 10 months into this lifestyle change and I'm not sure how I'll feel in a year or two about this indulgence described above. Should I be setting an example of what eating clean looks like? Will my friends feel more apt to make wise decisions for themselves if they see someone else doing so? Do I appear to be hypocritical to my friends who see that I'm not just eating plant-based foods? I'm still not totally clear on this subject but I know for sure it's not my place to challenge people personally who are not ready to make changes leading to greater health.

Chapter 12

The Struggle

There is no doubt, there will be a struggle. It's not easy to change, but it is possible. However, I don't see how it's possible to succeed without a serious commitment to the lifestyle.

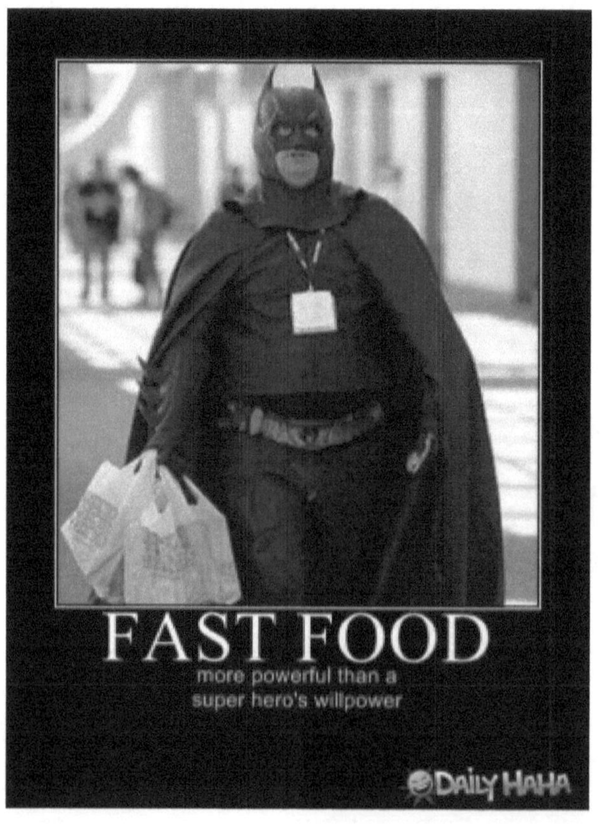

Even with a serious commitment and powerful motivation, most people will have occasional setbacks and slip ups. That's OK as long as you don't make a habit of them. Just get back on track, forget the mistake or indulgence and remind yourself why you are making these changes. It's a good idea to have a 3x5 card in your possession at all times with some motivating words or quotes. Keep it in your wallet or purse and pull it out whenever you are tempted. Below are some sample ideas to get you started. Write a few of your own and keep that card in your possession at all times. Copy them out of the book and take them with you everywhere.

My Health Goals Are Important to Me

- I want to be healthy and have the energy to keep up with my children and or grandchildren.
- I want to feel my best physically every day, be disease free and free of all prescription medications and their harmful side effects.
- I want to feel great every day and eating right makes that possible.
- I want to take control of my health.
- I have self-control that leads to higher self-esteem and better outcomes.
- I want to have the power and energy to spare that comes from eating healthy plant-based foods.
- I love my new lifestyle and I love eating nutritious food.

- I have proved that I am a powerful human being and I make decisions that benefit myself and my family.
- Nothing is more important than my health . . . *nothing!*
- I'm a strong person and I make wise decisions regarding my health.

You get the idea. Write down the affirmations that will help you when you need a little inspiration as you pass though the chips, soda and cookies section of your supermarket. To struggle and overcome is all a part of this process. Again, *you can do this*. Two steps forward and one step back will get you where you want to go . . . eventually. Anyone can make the changes and improve their overall health. You need to stay positive to stick with it. There are plant-based support groups in almost every city and many on line to choose from. The internet can be a tremendous resource of information and motivation. Everything you'll need to succeed is waiting for you on Netflix, on YouTube, on Google or at the website I've created – www.ourpassionforhealth.org. It's all there. "Seek and you will find!" Remember, there is great truth and honesty involved in what you are doing, and you are doing the right thing. You must believe that it's going to be worth the effort, because it is. That is the truth and it will take you to a higher place in life mentally as well as physically.

Please don't misunderstand, I went through this myself and if I can do it, I believe anyone can. Nevertheless, I certainly struggled and had my setbacks. Here is a summary I cut and pasted directly from my food diary.

Summary from My Food Diary

May 27

It's been a while since I've visited this diary. I've been on the diet since 3/7. In March, I stopped drinking, ate mostly vegetables but went off the diet a few times. Once when I went camping, I drank alcohol and ate meat. And a few other times when my son, Josh, came to visit I ate restaurant food. But since April 1st, I've stayed almost 100% on the straight and narrow path all the time and did some partial fasting and no alcohol. In six weeks I was able to get off all my medications. I've been prescription drug free for about 10 days now. My blood pressure is questionable, I'm still a little high 130/80 to 140/80 while off my meds. Today, I was 120/80 after a long walk. I have added in a few "off the path" meals in the past week. That was one meal eaten at a restaurant but then I went right back to the basics. When I do eat out, I order mostly salads and maybe salmon. I've been eating avocados, salads, sweet potatoes, walnuts, and healthy smoothies with berries and green powders and bone protein etc. I have also added a piece of wild Alaskan salmon about once a week. I've also had a beer a couple times in the past two weeks, but I've been very careful not to have two drinks at a time. I don't miss the drinking at all and could skip it altogether except in a social situation when I might want to join in to fit in but keeping it to one drink makes me happy.

I've been asked, what happens when you find yourself at home at 8:30 at night and you get hungry for some chips or something along those lines. It's easy for me because I don't buy anything that isn't healthy. No chips, no ice-cream, nothing except healthy foods. I do have a few fruit snacks like grapes, figs and baked apples with raisins. That satisfies my sweet tooth. The key here is not to be tempted by anything in your home. If you don't want to eat it, don't buy it and keep it out of your home. If you have to go to the store and buy some chips or cookies, it will take some time to get your wallet, keys and get to the car and you'll have time to change your mind and get back on track. So far so good. No heartburn in months without Prilosec.

Good Results Leading to a Major Physical Setback

Oct 25
It's been 5 months since that last post and I've had a few setbacks since then. It's going to happen from time to time. I was very strict with myself the first 6 to 8 weeks while I was attempting to heal my gut. I called that the healing phase. As a result of making the necessary changes, I was able to get off all my medications. Once I saw that my blood pressure was in the normal range and I was

heartburn free and free of the prescription meds associated with those problems, I started to gradually go off my prednisone, which controlled the pain from PMR, my autoimmune disease. PMR was by far my biggest problem and necessitated taking prednisone, the drug with the most serious side effects. You have to titrate off slowly because your adrenals have been supplemented by the drug and they need to be brought back on board slowly. I went from 20mgs to 10mg, 5mg to 5mg every other day and then, at last, off! Done! Finished! Healed! My rheumatologist wanted me to take 3 months to get off the drug. I did it within 6 weeks of being on my new lifestyle and the plant-based diet. This result borders on miraculous. Why is this seeming "miracle" such a secret? Truth — *food can be your medicine!*

After being off all my prescription drugs for a period of about two months, I started to feel amazing and totally like my younger active self again. As a result, I felt I was healed and after a few months I slowly began to slide back into my old patterns of eating and drinking. For example, I went to a deli and had my favorite sandwich . . . hot pastrami and I had been drinking a bit more. Then I had a three day mega physical experience that put a lot of pressure on my body. On Friday I had engaged in a hard-physical workout at the gym. I played basketball, I lifted weights and went for a swim. On Saturday, I participated in a major mountain bike ride. The ride was bumpy and jarring on my body. Sunday, I played golf. On Monday, I woke up feeling a little pain in my shoulders, which was to be expected considering the strenuous activity of the past three days. But the pain increased with each passing day until about two weeks later when I was suffering enough to pull out my left-over prednisone medication to put out the fire. I then went back to disciplined eating, as before. Two months later, back on the healthy lifestyle, I was off the prednisone again and, as of this writing, I'm still drug free. I have kept to my healthy lifestyle for the most part — probably 90% of the time, meaning I'll have a beer once in a while and eat the dinner my friends prepare and serve me, but that's about it. I like being healthy and drug free! Mindfulness: How am I feeling?

Mindfulness

Mindfulness is a popular topic these days. Mindfulness, when applied to eating can be very helpful in discovering what foods work best for your body. Mindfulness is a mental state achieved by focusing one's conscious awareness on the moment at hand, while calmly acknowledging and accepting one's feelings, thoughts, and bodily sensations present in that moment. We are all a little different in our chemistry makeup so it's important to watch what you eat and to be aware of this connection between what you eat and how you feel as a result. Most people don't recognize that connection. It could be that we become accustomed to feeling a certain way, a way that is not optimum, but the feeling is something we are used to and thus ignore. We may become drowsy after a big meal of meat and potatoes, but we think "that's to be expected" and we dismiss the connection or simply ignore it. We may experience "brain fog" after eating a large helping of sugar laden deserts. If your lunch salads get a good dose of dressing, it may be one of the causes of your brain fog. The food additive monosodium glutamate (MSG), used as a taste enhancer and flavoring agent, is hidden in almost all processed foods, ranging from bottled salad dressings, soups, and canned goods to many restaurant meals. People can experience physical symptoms when eating foods that contain MSG that last from a few hours to days, and the most common of these is brain fog. For those of you who are interested, here's how the chemistry works:

- Free glutamic acid is the active component in MSG and is converted to glutamate in the body.
- Glutamate is a neurotransmitter, or simply a chemical messenger, that transmits signals between neurons in the brain. However, too much glutamate is toxic to the brain as it triggers an excitotoxic state that leads to cell death.
- In addition, *glutamate overload depletes glutathione* and other powerful antioxidants that are needed to scavenge free radicals (toxic cellular waste) in the body. Sounds bad, right? It *is* bad.

There are lots of food-like-substances that have the potential to cause discomfort in your body and brain. *Pay attention to what makes you feel good and alive and focus on those foods. Avoid foods that seem to be holding you back and depleting your energy.* There is some conscious awareness needed to get this mix of foods just right, but you can do it. Anyone who cares enough to consciously pay attention to their health and is willing to make a few meaningful changes, based on mindfulness, will see immediate improvement in overall health — guaranteed!

A Food Diary

A food diary can be helpful in getting this mindfulness concept working for you. I started a food diary to document what seemed to be working and what was giving me problems. You might find this helpful on your journey back to health. Here is an example of my food diary along with a few guiding remarks and tips.

March 25th, 2018

(Three weeks after I started.)

8 am - feeling great! Got up and had a green smoothie. (Spinach, Kale and Chard, all organic greens, grabbed out of the bag and stuffed into my vita mix blender, with two cups of water and a little protein power. Hit the high-power button and it's ready in less than two minutes. Easy and quick and loaded with nutritious healing power.)

2 pm - ate a fresh avocado with Bragg's Vinaigrette made with organic apple cider vinegar. Delicious and nutritious. (Note: I wasn't a big avocado fan until I changed my habits. I found out that avocadoes are very healthy foods loaded with nutrition and especially known for providing the good fats – Omega 3s. I can eat almost anything if I know it's healthy and good for my body. I'm learning to like healthy foods and that's a good thing. It's my belief that most people, when they give this lifestyle a chance, will like and eventually love healthy foods more than they can imagine.)

7pm - I'm not really hungry so I ate an organic apple and that was it.

April 26th, 2018
8:15 am - Feeling great. Started the day off with a fruit smoothie. (Mostly frozen organic blueberries, cup of almond milk and some various health powers like protein power and bone broth powder and some spirulina type green powder. All into the blender, providing instant goodness. (Again, it takes no more than 3 minutes to get this drink made, very easy and filled with good stuff. Now I make enough to last a couple of days, so I have it handy whenever I need a quick pick me up.)

11:15 am - Fresh avocado mixed with a tomato and the vinaigrette dressing above. (Sometimes I'll add olives, or humus to the mix and it's all delicious and nutritious.)

3pm - A friend brought over a piece of his birthday cake. I ate it. <u>I felt a little tired afterwards. Sugar, I should have known better</u>.

6 pm - I ate a piece of wild salmon with lemon. Ate some raw carrots and had a baked apple for dessert. (I personally made the choice to add wild salmon to my healthy diet. I wanted to add the extra protein and the healthy fish oil, omega 3. Some may want to cut out all animal meats, even oily fish. It's up to you.)

The Bottom Line

Keeping a food diary can be helpful and is recommended especially during the first 6 to 8 weeks. After eleven months, I've created a new lifestyle for myself and I don't feel a need to write in my food diary as much but when I do, I keep it simple. I remember to take notes when something changes, or when I get a reaction from some part of my diet. That is, I'll note the brain fog, tiredness or lack of energy and record what food or habit caused the change.

Chapter 13

Exercise! Just do it!

Our focus up to now has been on diet and lifestyle and its importance in restoring one's health, but it's impossible to talk about superior health without addressing the utmost importance of maintaining a regular exercise program of some kind.

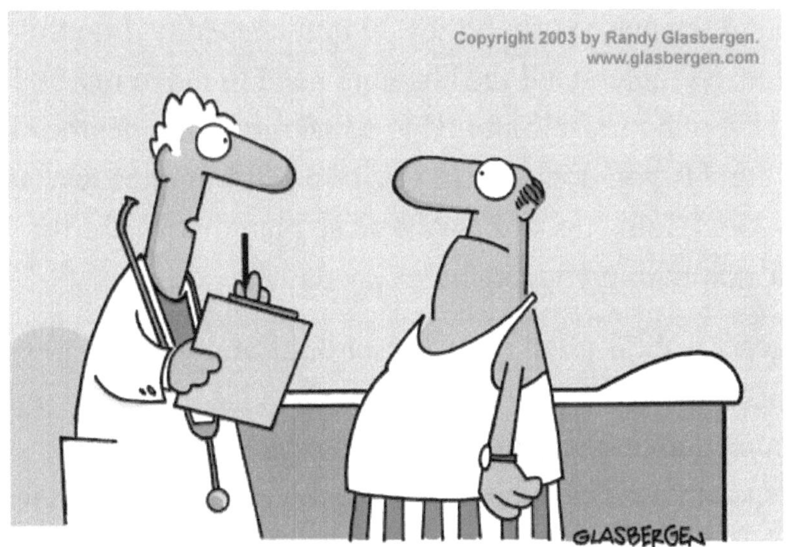

"What fits your busy schedule better, exercising one hour a day or being dead 24 hours a day?"

You may have this aspect of your life covered, if so, that's great, you can skip over this section. If not, read on. The good news is that it doesn't take hours in the gym to be healthy and fit. Studies have shown that a simple, daily routine of a twenty to thirty-minute walk will suffice. The benefits of getting regular exercise are too numerous to list here, but regular exercise is unquestionably a must if you want to live with a healthy body. Exercise will boost your energy, improve your muscle strength and boost your endurance. Exercise delivers oxygen and nutrients to your tissues and helps your cardiovascular system work more efficiently. When your heart and lung health improve, you will have more energy to tackle daily projects. I'm not a gym guy. It's just too boring for me, but I do enjoy walking around the neighborhood for 30 minutes a day. I do this because I understand the absolute need to move my body and keep my muscles toned to some minimum degree. The saying, "If you don't use it, you'll lose it," applies to your muscles. Come up with an exercise plan that works for you, something you can do every day.

When I walk, I often wear my earbuds and listen to music on Pandora or books on audible.com. This keeps my mind occupied and makes the time go by faster and usually extends my walks, which is good. When I go to the store or the mall, I purposely park in the outer edges of the parking lot. You get more room for your automobile and you get a chance to take a short walk. Every bit helps.

Two Great Benefits of Exercise

For those who are new to the scientifically proven benefits of exercise, here are some specific things you can expect if you take the time to get out of the house or office and move your body:
Exercise Reduces Your Risk for Serious Illness

Exercise reduces people's chances of developing and dying of illnesses such as heart disease. It does this by lowering illness risk factors such as triglyceride and overall cholesterol levels, while improving the level of HDL (the "good" cholesterol, which is thought to reduce the risk of heart disease). Weight-bearing exercise and strength training activities help to maintain or increase bone mass, reducing a person's risk for osteoarthritis and associated bone fractures. Regular exercise also lowers resting blood pressure rates for hours after an exercise session is over. In addition, moderate exercise may significantly reduce the risk of developing type II diabetes. Arthritics who exercise often experience more strength and flexibility in their affected joints as well as reduced pain levels. Furthermore, exercise may delay or prevent the development of arthritis in other joints. Regular walking of over a mile a day has been shown to reduce the risk of stroke significantly. Exercise even appears to reduce the risk of developing some cancers, especially cancers of the breast and colon.

A Real Plus: Exercise Increases Energy and Feelings of Vitality

Sedentary individuals often complain of being too tired to work out. Ironically, exercise improves people's capacity for work so that people who exercise on a regular basis actually have more energy and greater strength and endurance for daily activities than do their sedentary peers. The feeling of increased energy, and vitality is one of the first things people tend to notice a few weeks after beginning to work out on a regular basis. As Martha Stewart would say, "That's a very good thing."

I can only assume that you are reading this book because you want to restore your health and become uber healthy, right? Then you probably already know that it's impossible to be healthy without regular exercise. If not, you certainly know now. No excuses. It's an absolute must. Get up, get out and get moving!

Chapter 14

Knowledge = Power To Change

I believe that knowledge is power and that applies especially to your health. When you have the knowledge, you have the power to heal. How miraculous is that? It was self-education that created the spark of belief inside me and it was that spark that brought about the change I needed personally. I started by watching Netflix food-nutrition-oriented documentaries and that worked for me. They were interesting and informative. I can't stress enough the value of searching out health, food and plant-based documentaries as an easy place to start. Below are a few to look for. There are many more out there and more on the way all the time. Find the ones that spark your food revolution. By the way, you are now a part of the vanguard of health-minded people that is slowly but surely changing the world . . . one bite at a time. Here are some of my favorite food-nutrition based documentaries to look for:

Food Documentaries

- *Forks Over Knives*
- *Hungry for Change*
- *Rotten*
- *Food Choices*

- *Food Inc.*
- *In Defense of Food*
- *Prescription Thugs*

May I also suggest going to YouTube and putting into the search bar: "wholefood plant-based diet" and "plant-based healing" and watch any number of personal testimonials and lectures from individuals and doctors explaining the benefits of the plant-based lifestyle. In fact, whenever you are feeling weak and slipping away from what you know is right, YouTube health videos can be a great source of motivation and inspiration. I highly recommend them in those moments of doubt. If you prefer to read your information, Amazon has many books on living the plant-based lifestyle. I stress that there is a world of information and help and encouragement all around us. Take advantage of it, and remember what Winston Churchill said to his people during WWII: *"Never give up! Never give up! Never give up!" And they didn't give up and they won the war and so can you!*

Once you have the knowledge and the power that comes with it, you'll be in a better position to make drastic changes in favor of your health and you'll see positive results on every side. Not only will you see the positive side of experiencing better health, but that positive step will create new pathways in the brain and create a feeling of self-control and self-empowerment. That leads to a new belief system that enlightens one's vision for the future and brightens one's path to a greater experience in life, which leads to happiness.

Am I saying that eating a plant-based diet is a panacea? Yes, exactly! I contend that when you make the change to a healthy, clean, plant-based lifestyle, it will simultaneously improve all the other areas of one's life as well, making you a healthier AND happier individual.

Nothing, *absolutely nothing* is more important to your overall well-being and happiness than getting as healthy as you possibly can. Everything else in your life will improve because of it! Without good health, everything else in life is handicapped in one way or another. Do yourself a great favor and *get healthy!*

Imagine you won the lottery and spent over a hundred thousand dollars on your dream car — for me that might be a new Porsche 911 Carrera. Now, you have the car, it's yours, it goes from 0-60mph in 4.2 seconds and you love it. You go out to the garage and look at it from time to time and think how lucky and fortunate you are to have this great machine with the amazing stereo etc. If your dream car called for high-test gasoline, you wouldn't put regular gas in it, would you? You wouldn't drive it around needing a tune up, would you? No! You'd put the high-octane fuel it called for and keep the car properly tuned and running at its best. Of course, your body is worth way more than any Porsche and your own body is much more important to your overall level of happiness than any dream car could ever be.

By getting your body and mind in the best possible condition through proper eating habits and regular exercise, you'll be able to face the world with your best foot forward. Feeling powerful in body and mind is a necessity in the competitive, fast-paced world we live in today. Being in the best shape possible health-wise will give us the edge we need. Why waste the vast human potential inherent in your being? You may never know what that is until you go to the next level in your health, reaching and stretching out for that promised land. Don't doubt it for a second, the promised land of vitality and health is there waiting for you.

The point here is this: there needs to be a new awareness of the importance of being healthy. I want to plant this fact firmly plant in your mind. There is immense value in being the healthiest you can be. I want people to see the importance of taking full control of their health. You have the ability to gain that control. It's about so much more than just eating a plant-based diet. It's about the new, stronger, more enlightened person you'll become by taking the journey from ignorance and dissipation to knowledge and wisdom-based eating and living. The new lifestyle creates a better and stronger person health-wise. Just as importantly, it improves your outlook on the world and your place in it. It's empowering on so many levels, and who doesn't want more power in their lives? Everyone does! That is my goal, to empower people to take the path less traveled that leads to greater health and to a greater life in general. ***When you find a person who is passionate about their health, you'll find a person who is passionate about their life!***

Don't get me wrong, there is a price to pay before this change can take place. Giving up habits and changing your lifestyle does not come easy. The proposition needs to be fully understood before taking the leap. You need to believe that the work involved in making this change is going to be worth it. That is a vital purpose of this book. I want to explain the proposition in a way that makes it crystal clear that the benefits are great and numerous in comparison to the price you pay. It's like the "pearl of great price" that Jesus talked about:

> "Again, the kingdom of heaven
> is like unto a merchant man,
> seeking goodly pearls: Who,
> when he had found one pearl of
> great price, went and sold all that
> he had, and bought it."

Matthew 13:45–46, King James Version

Finding the "pearl of great price" is like discovering the innate value in eating right and becoming vital and healthy. There is truly nothing more important to you than your health. If you don't believe me, just ask a sick rich man what he'd pay to be well again, for what good is

133

money if you have no vitality to enjoy it? You need health and vitality to enjoy most of what is available to a human being on this planet.

Once you realize the value of making the change, nothing will stand in your way and no price will be too much to receive what you'll get by taking control of your own health! You just need to believe it will be worth it. Believe it! It is worth it! Keep in mind the popular saying: **Health is the New Wealth!** And everyone wants to be wealthy, right?

Unlike the pearl of great price, getting healthy is easy to obtain. You don't have to sell "all your goods" but you do need to give up some or all of your limiting bad habits. How can you do that? You just have to see and appreciate the great and undeniable value of living a healthy lifestyle. How can I get there? Keep reading and watching and listening to plant-based truth, and continue to educate yourself, and then go for it like your life depends on it. Once you see and understand the true value of taking control of your health, then making "health" your top priority is easy. You will have no problem committing to the process of positive change when you know in your heart and mind that it's going to be worth it. Getting healthy is the *pearl of great price* of your life. You learn what is important to your body and you provide it. You are the gatekeeper of your mouth and only you can properly feed it. Taking control of your health is literally one of the wisest and smartest decisions you have the opportunity to make in life. Please, for your own sake, make that decision before it's too late.

Control is a Key Concept!

This concept cannot be overstated. There are many forces present in your life that are totally out of your control. These uncontrollable forces can and do affect what happens to you today and in your future, but eating is not one of those things! With eating, you are the only one that's in charge. Isn't that great! No one can force you to make bad food choices. Ultimately, you have no one to blame but yourself for your poor health decisions as they relate to lifestyle choices.

And . . . you have no one to thank but yourself. You can take full credit for the journey and adventure you have chosen, and you will personally benefit from all the many blessings you'll receive. Bring all the truth to bear. We can get off drugs if we want to. We can be healthy if we want to. It's as simple as being careful of what goes into your piehole (hopefully, not pie). It's easy once you've made the movement in the right direction. The momentum toward healthy living pulls you forward with constant positive reinforcement because you are walking in the truth and the truth is setting you free. This is still a revelation and a revolution in the way we think about eating.

Chapter 15

Diet vs. Lifestyle

What is the first thing you think of when you think of diet? Exactly . . . "Diets don't work!" Diets are perceived as temporary and rarely work.

According to the American Council of Exercise, only five percent of dieters are able to successfully keep the weight off after dieting. Most dieters regain a third of the weight within one year of going off the diet and gain back almost all the weight they lost within three to five years. I found this interesting as I was searching out the meaning of "diet". The word *diet* first appeared in English in the 13th century. Its original meaning was the same as in modern English, "habitually taken food and drink." But *diet* was used in another sense too in the Middle and early modern English periods to mean "way of living." This is, in fact, the original meaning of *diet*'s Greek ancestor *diaita,* which is derived from the verb *diaitasthan,* meaning "to lead one's life." In Greek, *diaita,* had already come to be used more specifically for a way of living prescribed by a physician.

I like the original Greek meaning: "to lead one's life". That sounds like one's diet is the core and guiding principal in their lives. The Diet is the leader, the guide, the determiner. So, putting yourself on a diet could be a good thing. After all, a diet is the first step toward a lifestyle change, right?

Most nutritionists suggest that changing your lifestyle is more efficient and healthier than just dieting for a short period. A diet is a systematized, temporary change, whereas changing one's lifestyle is an attempt to keep up similar habits for a prolonged period of time — for a lifetime, in fact.

A lifestyle, once embraced, is a chosen way of life . . . for life, and once on that path, it has staying power. A lifestyle includes what you eat, how you manage stress, how much you exercise and more. Lifestyle changes require you to maintain a certain level of dieting and restricting how much fast food and junk food you eat, etc., but there are not as many restrictions placed on it. If you succumb to temptation here and there, it's not the end of the world. You are aware and might feel a little bit of quilt, but are still in touch with your actions without completely giving up. It's very important to remember that moderation is the key to maintaining a healthy lifestyle without depriving yourself of things you want to have once in a while.

The small percentage of people who've regained and maintained their good health over several years have made true lifestyle changes. That's the key to success, not adherence to fad diets. **Lifestyle changes aren't**

temporary. If you follow a precise low-glycemic plan, stop for a month, go back to your old habits, and then start up again, you're not really making changes to your lifestyle.

We all know that unhealthy lifestyles lead to a long list of ailments and diseases that are eventually too uncomfortable to be tolerated and at that point we may do something about it or continue to suffer and die an agonizing premature death. It's your choice. Life or Death.

Think: the undisciplined lifestyle generally leads to an overweight condition that is unhealthy. The individual, if they care about themselves at all, will eventually make the difficult decision to "go on a diet". If successful in the short term, they lose the weight and are happy with themselves and then slowly go back to what they were doing in the past and the unhealthy lifestyle reemerges along with the excess weight.

The problem is simple. They are changing their diet when they should be changing their lifestyle.

Lifestyle Changes are all About Balance

Discovering balance is the key to making long-term changes work. Without balance, you can wind up feeling deprived and defeated, or even overwhelmed with the need to be perfect. Know that there'll be times when flexibility is the name of the game and allow yourself to indulge without losing your focus.

- **Lifestyle changes become a natural part of your routine.** In the beginning, trying to lose weight, for example, requires some focus as you find ways to incorporate low-glycemic foods (foods that don't spike your insulin as much as others) and cut back on the number of overall calories you consume. Yet eventually the new actions you're taking (such as diet changes and exercise) turn into a habit.

 (*Note:* You may need to switch up your strategies once in a while if your current path isn't working well in your lifestyle.)

- **Lifestyle changes must be things you can do on your own.** Following someone else's plan is only a temporary fix. Doing over the long-term would be truly difficult due to the loss of personal preference and choice. Figuring out how to plan healthy meals on your own is the more realistic option.

When you know how to plan your meals, you can plan healthy eating anytime, anywhere, whether you're on vacation or at the office.

*"Men's natures are alike; it is their habits that separate them." – **Confucius***

LIFESTYLE! Key Idea:

Most people are living a lifestyle that they grew into without giving it much thought. They may have hung out with a certain class or type of people in high school, the party crowd, drinking to excess and doing recreational drugs and they simply continued that lifestyle into adulthood. They are in the habit of doing certain things on the weekend and don't really think about it. It could be said they are living the "party lifestyle". Many continue this to the extreme until they develop an addiction to a substance that ruins their life. And that's the problem. *Not thinking.* Most lifestyles are simply habits that we develop as young adults and continue for years, again without much thought. It's only when these habits hinder our progress that one begins to reflect and think of making changes. A healthy lifestyle, unless you are lucky, doesn't develop naturally and is a lifestyle you must consciously choose and usually unless one becomes sick there is little impetus to examine one's course in life or see the need for change. How much better we'd all be if we examined the various lifestyles available to us and chose a lifestyle that gave us the best opportunity for living the best life possible. That's what this section is about, making a wise choice regarding which direction we'd like to go in life and choosing a lifestyle that will get us there.

If you are suffering from a chronic disease, are taking numerous prescriptions, have high blood pressure, autoimmune disease, chronic fatigue syndrome or any other conditions where you believe you are being held back in life because of your ill health, then perhaps it's time to take a look at your lifestyle and see how that is affecting your body. The core message of this book is: **Choosing to embrace the healthy lifestyle is vital to experiencing a more rewarding life**. We need to understand the importance of making a lifestyle change. This is a big step but a necessary step in the process of getting well and staying well and becoming your best self. You must see yourself reborn as a healthy-minded individual.

Chapter 16.

Bridging the Gap and Taking the Leap

Right now, take a minute to relax, take a deep breath and envision yourself as a healthy person, a person who does healthy things and acts in healthy ways. See yourself eating healthy plant-based food and loving it. See yourself exercising and loving it. See yourself as the picture of pristine health with a glow on your cheeks and a bounce in your step. Think about it, visualize it. Make this change in perception of yourself to get to the other side of the equation. You must believe you can do it and it's going to be worth whatever the perceived cost or whatever effort you may deem necessary. It's imperative! But how?

Visualize and totally identify yourself first and foremost as a healthy individual. This is an underlying principal. If you've read this far, you've seen the light. You know you want to live life to the fullest and you know that being a healthy person is the first step in making that happen. The first goal here is to get to the place where you understand. Understand what? You understand that your body is your most valuable and important possession and it makes sense to cherish your body above all things. You can see now that doing so is wisdom personified. You know this deep in your soul. You understand this wisdom. You just need to give it some thought and some time and take appropriate action to turn these ideas and concepts into a lifestyle — your new lifestyle. But how can I make this leap of faith from where I am now to this promised land you are describing, where I'm healthier and happier?

The Three Steps

I have an idea that might bridge the gap…you need to get…

From: *"This sounds good, positive and interesting, but I don't think I can make that leap,"* or *"I love my fried foods too much"*, *"I love my cigarettes,"* or *I love my . . . (fill in the blank)*______________ and *"I'm not sure if I can do it."*

To: *"This is great and awesome for me. This is what I've been looking for. This is totally doable. I'm doing this! I'll set the example! I'll be drug free and disease free and have more energy than I know what to do with! I'm changing my lifestyle to a positive health-style. "*

If that sounds good and where you really want to be, may I suggest you embrace the following three steps:

Before you begin, find a quiet place where you won't be disturbed and grab a notepad. OK, ready? All quiet? Then let's go for it. Read the following, in quotations, like your life depends on it . . . because it does.

Step One: Recognition of the Problem

"I realize that I have taken my health for granted. I've paid little attention to what I've been putting into my mouth. I know now that I can do better to feel better."

Think about it deeply right now for a few minutes until you feel this truth in your soul. It's OK to feel a little regret knowing that you could have paid more attention to something as important as your health but didn't until now. That was then. Now you are aware and you realize that your health _is_ the most important thing in your life and you are giving it the priority it deserves! When you get this understanding in your heart and soul, then go to Step Two. Otherwise, keep thinking about it until you feel it and get it.)

Step Two: Affirmation of your life

 With the new understanding from Step One, and with feeling in your heart, say the following . . .

> "Right now, on this day, in this
> moment I realize that _Life is
> Beautiful_, and I want to live the
> rest of my life to the fullest, and
> make the most of it. I want to
> experience my full potential as a

> human being. I want to be
> vibrant and filled with energy
> and feel my best every day. I'm
> aware of and thankful for the
> amazing life I've been given. I
> want to make the most of it
> starting with living a vibrant and
> healthy lifestyle."

Think about it. Really! Stop, look within yourself and contemplate your future life. You've been given this gift of life on planet Earth. The least you can do is to take good care of yourself beginning with your body! Feel it. Do you want to give back? Say *"Yes! Staying healthy is my moral responsibility for the gift of life I've received. **Never again will I be wasteful with my health"***. Doesn't this make sense? Say "Yes," to the healthy lifestyle for the rest of your life. Are we getting this? Think about it. What could be better or make more sense?

Step Three: Repentance

Repentance: the activity of reviewing one's actions and feeling contrition or regret for past wrongs, which is accompanied by commitment to change for the better.

Are you there yet? Are you feeling it? Are you seeing it? If not, go back to the previous steps and think more about it as it relates to YOU and the best of all possible worlds — for you! Are we getting it? Got it? Good! OK, let's move forward with Step Three . . . read, think and be as you say the following:

"I acknowledge that I have not done my part to keep my health a top priority. I've suffered in ignorance and paid a dear price for my harmful and self-destructive ways, but now I know better! I've obtained wisdom and knowledge in this area, I'm now I'm *empowered* and realize that I have the intelligence and **inner strength** to change my bad habits and create new ones that will lead to my greater experience in life. I realize the utmost value of changing my lifestyle to a positive *health style*. For me, it's about health in every way! I'm moving forward to becoming the best healthy person I can be. I choose to be wiser now, today and every day. **I forgive and forget my ignorance of the past. I simply didn't know what I was doing.** But now I know what to do and how to do it. Now I give my life a higher value and I understand there is a better, much better way to eat and live and be. I identify with health. I am my healthiest and happiest self and I do my part in making the right choices every day, as best I can. I am a new person. I am a healthy person. I live in a healthy environment. I personify health in everything I do. People see me as a great example of a person who cares. I see myself as a strong, disciplined and loving person, totally capable of achieving anything I put my mind to. I have mastered the key to health, and I've opened the door. I am the master of my own health and wellbeing. I am already on this straight and narrow path that leads to my best self and my best life. I've begun my journey to health. I am consciously aware this day, this moment in time that I have the power to change and I am now embracing this new idea of myself. I am happy now that I have taken the road less traveled that leads me into a true adventure story — a story where I am the hero. I know now that I want to be a healthy person and I want to live a healthy lifestyle for the rest of my life . . . **<u>Let the Adventure Begin!</u>**

Your signature_____________________________________

date of your personal rebirth ___________________ (In the space below, write what you are feeling right now along with your own inspirational thoughts.)

Notes continued:

And may I suggest:

*If you are a person who believes in prayer, pray for the strength to be the hero of your own personal adventure story.

*If you are a meditator or into yoga, meditate on the above three steps, and say, "OOOOMMM!"

*If you are an agnostic, think about learning more about yourself and how taking the three steps might actually work for you. Think about how cool it would be to do this, as an experiment in your life. Believe that the steps will work for you and bring you closer to the goal of pristine health and know that's just the start of great new beginnings for you. Focus on that positive thought . . . Believe it, a change, a good change is coming!

*If you are a die-hard, card-carrying atheist, and you really believe that there is no greater intelligence out there than yours, then make being uber healthy your god . . . I mean Goal, and step into the new healthy lifestyle. You'll be glad you did but only if you have the discipline to master this key to good health.

Chapter 17

What Should I Eat to Get Started?

Now that you are in the place where you want to be your healthiest self, your best self, you might be asking, "How do I get moving in the right direction?" It was suggested that I map out a detailed list of what I'd recommend eating when first getting started on this new lifestyle. It was at that moment that I realized I'm not much of a cook. I have chosen what's easy for me. That might be too bland for others. The following is what I ate over the first 7 days of my new lifestyle *diet*. If you are a "foodie" and like to cook, you can easily improve on my feeble, first-week meal plan. If you are as clueless as I was, the detailed notes from my food diary might be of help to get you started. I've added some discussion notes to the 7-day diary on topics that I was curious about or struggled with and did research on to determine which way I should go. I hope you'll find these notes helpful.

What I need to make perfectly clear is that if you are attempting to be free of your diseases and eliminate the prescription drugs you are currently taking, you'll need to stick to organic fresh fruits and vegetables for a period of 6 to 8 weeks. That's not really very long compared to taking drugs for years. So, that means no sugar, no bread, no meat except occasional fish dishes like salmon, no dairy . . . again, just fresh organic fruits and vegetables. If it comes in a box, skip it. Some would consider this quite restrictive, but you still have the entire world of fruits and vegetables to choose from which is a lot of choices. Let's use our imagination.

After you are disease free you may decide to bring in other foods to add variety to your menu. If you want to have an occasional steak, make sure the beef is grass fed and free of antibiotics — if its grass fed it should be. If you are craving a piece of pizza, enjoy . . . once in a while. This all comes down to lifestyle. Living a lifestyle means you know what you are doing. You are eating healthy to be healthy, and you are aware of the pitfalls of eating non-nutritious foods so you don't make them a habit. The point is, to maintain a healthy lifestyle, you need to make wise choices 80 to 90 percent of the time. If you are doing that, you'll be happy and healthy. The difficult one to overcome is sugar-laden foods. Cookies, bread, ice cream, cakes, pies etc. The problem with sugar is that, when you eat it, it creates a craving for more of the same and it's hard not to get sucked back into a downward sugar cycle of death. So, think of sugar as poison. If in doubt, reread the chapter on sugar.

As you can see, going on a diet means more than just restricting one's self to certain foods but that's a big part of it.

Let's face it, the road to a healthy lifestyle begins with diet. The key is to understand the big picture. Remind yourself always of the vital reasons why you entertained the thought of this health concept in the first place. You need to know what you are doing and why you are doing it. And in doing so, you are demonstrating wisdom to yourself, your family and to your community. Be happy because you are wiser now. You made this decision to change your lifestyle because you thought deeply about the matter of your health and you came to the correct conclusions:

1. That being healthy is important to you and your family.
2. That you have done your own due diligence regarding the way you want to eat and live . . . (reading this book is certainly part of that)
3. And now you know better — you know that the healthy lifestyle is the best option for you and all concerned.

I'm going to lay out some easy-to-follow meal choices and show you how to prepare meals that will get you started on the right foot.

Preliminary Step: Give away or throw out anything in your pantry or fridge that is not going to be a part of your new healthy lifestyle. You don't want to be wasteful so bag it up and give it to the local homeless. Manufactured foods, sweets of any kind, breads, most things that come in a box and have a long shelf life, cola, and anything else you know is not part of your new healthy life needs to go. Once you start on this health journey, you don't want to be tempted with sweets and processed foods that will set you back. Helpful hint: load up on fruits and nuts to keep them handy. The time will come when you are craving sweets and you'll want to have ample real food substitutes that can satisfy you in a pinch. More on this latter.

Here is what I ate the first 7 days to get started.

Day 1.

Breakfast — Morning smoothie:

Put any kind of organic fruit, frozen or fresh, into the blender. I use frozen blue berries or a frozen berry blend from Costco. I use at least a cup of fruit and add a cup of water or almond milk and a scoop of protein power or other type of healthy "green" power to the mix and blend it for a minute or longer depending on your blender. I recommend investing in a Viti Mix. It is expensive but it will last forever and is the best on the market.

Hint: make enough to cover you for a couple of days. Put the left-over smoothie in a large plastic container and take it with you to work if you have access to a fridge there.

Lunch:

Avocado with any healthy oil-based dressing you prefer. If still hungry, eat two avocados. You can always add any vegetables to the meal.

Dinner:

Sweet potato with olive oil and raisins for sweetness. Sometimes I pour a little olive oil or dressing on the potato if it's too dry. (more on dressings later)

Day 2.

Breakfast: Bowl of old fashioned or steel cut oatmeal with fruit. (Not the instant, processed kind of oatmeal — but you already knew that, didn't you?) I like grape raisins or cranberry raisins. I put them into the bowl with water or almond milk and cook them along with the oatmeal. Applesauce provides a good topping. I use my microwave because I like to make it quick and easy for myself. I'm eating in three minutes. I don't have to tell you how oatmeal sticks to your ribs and keeps you going all morning and into the afternoon.

Lunch: Avocados, one or two with Romaine lettuce, add the dressing of your choice . . . oil based, no store-bought creamy dressings, but you knew that already. If you are really hungry, add more lettuce, eat as much as you want, stuff yourself! It's all good. Also, I keep a large jar of Italian olives that I like and will put them on almost anything or eat them by themselves. Pick a variety of olives that you personally enjoy.

Dinner: Don't think of dinner as your "big" meal of the day, it's just another opportunity to feed your body what it needs to recover. I might just have a vegetable smoothie. (Smoothies are no longer just breakfast food!) I use water or almond milk as a base, then stuff the blender with green food of the leafy kind. Larger grocery stores these days carry a prepackaged bag of healthy greens. We're talking the kings and queens of the healthy leafy plants. Kale, Chard and spinach mostly. Blend it all together with a plant-based protein powder of some kind to give the drink more flavor . . . if you want to. You may love the taste of just the green juice smoothie without the added powder. It's up to you. If you want a beverage besides water, have a kombucha drink filled with healthful pro-biotics.

Desert: If, like myself, you get the urge for something sweet once in a while, here are some suggestions. Grapes of all kinds, Apple, Pear, plumb or cherry, banana, pineapple . . . whatever you want. What I came up with was a baked apple. Here's my recipe. Cut a fresh apple up into 4 pieces and put them into a microwaveable bowl face up, skin down. Sprinkle cinnamon all over the apples. Place your favorite raisins and a few slices of ripe bananas on top. Use as much toping as you like . . . more bananas, less raisins, add a different fruit that you may prefer. Put that into the microwave for 3 to 5 minutes and it comes out smelling delicious and you are going to love it. Sweet tooth averted.

Cinnamon is a favorite spice I use liberally on a lot of different foods and it has lots of health benefits. Cinnamon provides high amounts of calcium and fiber. One teaspoon provides a whopping 22% of the daily recommended value in manganese. What does manganese do for you? A lot, actually. Manganese is a trace mineral that helps the body form strong bones, connective tissues, and sex hormones. It also helps coagulate the blood properly. Manganese helps metabolize fat and carbohydrates, regulate blood sugar, absorb calcium, and is essential for optimal brain and nerve function. As if that's not enough, it's also a component of the antioxidant enzyme superoxide dismutase, which helps neutralize free radicals that can damage cell membranes and DNA. Proper levels of manganese have been linked to the prevention of diabetes, arthritis, epilepsy, and even PMS. There is also an antimicrobial effect that was known to the ancient Egyptians, who used cinnamon in their mummification processes.

According to a study, just smelling cinnamon or chewing cinnamon gum is enough to boost brain activity. In fact, test scores were higher, and memory, visual recognition, and motor speed were greatly enhanced in individuals who took a whiff of cinnamon, compared with individuals who smelled jasmine, peppermint, or no fragrance at all. So, there you have it. Buy a large jar of cinnamon and use it liberally.

Day 3.

Breakfast: Fruit smoothie (change up the fruits to keep it interesting).

Lunch: Veggie scramble. Eggs! I love eggs and they are so versatile. Let's talk about eggs and how they fit into a plant-based diet. Some say no eggs and others see value. Here are some thoughts:

There are two different camps. One lead by the "forks over knives" crew who recommend not eating eggs and have studies to back up their negative attitude. But first, let's see what the pro-egg folks have to say. Here is their argument:

Why Eat Eggs

If you're a vegetarian, then it's highly likely that you already appreciate the health benefits of eating a plant-based diet. Eating that way for health reasons means lower blood pressure and cholesterol levels, more stable blood sugar,
and a reduced incidence of cancer. That's above and beyond the other benefits, such as having more energy, clearer skin, and even the reversal of health-related conditions. However, some vegans stick to eating only those foods that are derived from the earth . . . with the exception of eggs, yes, they eat eggs.

What makes eggs such an important part of the diet that they've worked their way into a traditional plant-based lifestyle? As it turns out, there are three pretty solid reasons.

Top 3 Reasons to Eat Eggs

1. Higher Energy Levels
Eggs have long been considered one of the best protein sources available, with each one supplying roughly 6 grams. Protein is critical not only for helping your body build muscle mass, but also for giving you enough energy to get through your busy day.

This reason is probably more important today than ever before as it seems like we're always running from one thing to the next with little time to just sit and relax.

In this way, eating eggs essentially helps give you that *oomph* you need to accomplish all of the amazing things you want to do.

Tweet: "If you've broken the eggs, you should make the omelet ~ Anthony Eden"

2. Eat Eggs to Losing or Maintaining Weight
Have you ever noticed that you have an easier time waiting for lunch when you eat eggs for breakfast than when you choose other options like cereal or a bagel? Again, this is due largely to the protein in eggs, a result which makes it

easier to lose weight or, if you're already where you want to be, maintain a healthy weight.

3. Greater Health

One of the reasons a plant-based diet is so good for you is because of the many different vitamins and minerals it provides, ultimately giving you a higher level of health. Well, the same is true when it comes to eggs, because they contain a number of healthy nutrients as well. They include vitamins A, B2, B5, and B12; along with phosphorus, selenium, iron, choline, and a variety of amino acids.

Eggs also supply your body with a good dose of two different antioxidants, specifically lutein and zeaxanthine. These have been linked with greater eye health, reducing your risk of macular degeneration or cataracts.

If I eat eggs won't my cholesterol levels increase? Amidst all of these benefits, the concern most people have when it comes to eggs is cholesterol. However, reputable health agencies like the <u>Mayo Clinic</u> indicate that the cholesterol in eggs has very little effect on blood cholesterol levels. The only exception is for diabetics, as eggs can increase the risk of heart disease for this portion of the population.

How to Incorporate Eggs in Your Diet

If you are considering going vegan to enjoy these types of benefits, you can incorporate eggs into your diet fairly easily. For instance, you can poach them, scramble them, or fry them in a little heart-healthy olive oil and have a filling breakfast. You can also add them later in the day and a hard-boiled egg packs nicely for a hike.

Forks over Knives Official Argument:

A common question I hear is, "What's wrong with eggs?" (Second only to "Where do you get your protein?")

Where to begin? Let's start with the obvious egg facts. Eggs have zero dietary fiber, and about 70 percent of their calories are from fat — a big portion of which is saturated. They are also loaded with cholesterol — about 213 milligrams for an average-sized egg. For reference, people with diabetes, cardiovascular disease, or high cholesterol should consume fewer than 200 milligrams of cholesterol each day. (Uh oh.) And, humans have no biological need to consume any cholesterol at all; we make more than enough in our own bodies.

Why so much fat and cholesterol in such a tiny package? Think about it: eggs hold every piece of the puzzle needed to produce a new life. Within that shell lies the capacity to make feathers, eyes, a beak, a brain, a heart, and so on. It takes a lot of stuff to make such a complex being.

In addition to these excessive (for humans) natural components of an egg, other human-health hazards exist. Because eggshells are fragile and porous, and conditions on egg farms are crowded, eggs are the perfect host for salmonella — the leading cause of food poisoning in the U.S.

How Eggs Affect Us

Those are some facts and figures. But how do eggs affect real people in real life? Luckily, researchers have conducted good studies to help answer that question.

Cancer

In a 1992 analysis of dietary habits, people who consumed just 1.5 eggs per week had nearly five times the risk for colon cancer, compared with those who consumed hardly any (fewer than 11 per year), according to the *International Journal of Cancer*. The World Health Organization analyzed data from 34 countries in 2003 and found that eating eggs is associated with death from colon and rectal cancers. And a 2011 study funded by the National Institutes of Health showed that eating eggs is linked to developing prostate cancer. By consuming 2.5 eggs per week, men increased their risk for a deadly form of prostate cancer by 81 percent, compared with men who consumed less than half an egg per week. Finally, even moderate egg consumption tripled the risk of developing bladder cancer, according to a 2005 study published in *International Urology and Nephrology*.

Diabetes

A review of fourteen studies published earlier this year in the journal *Atherosclerosis* showed that people who consumed the most eggs increased their risk for diabetes by 68 percent, compared with those who ate the fewest.

In a 2008 publication for the Physicians' Health Study I, which included more than 21,000 participants, researchers found that those who consumed seven or more eggs per week had an almost 25 percent increased risk of death compared to those with the lowest egg consumption. The risk of death for participants with diabetes who ate seven or more eggs per week was twice as high as for those who consumed the fewest number of eggs.

Egg consumption also increases the risk of gestational diabetes, according to two 2011 studies referenced in the *American Journal of Epidemiology*. Women who consumed the most eggs had a 77 percent increased risk of diabetes in one study and a 165 percent increased risk in the other, compared with those who consumed the least.

Heart Disease

Researchers published a blanket warning in the *Canadian Journal of Cardiology,* informing readers that ceasing egg consumption after a heart attack would be "a necessary act, but late." In the previously mentioned 14-study review, researchers found that people who consumed the most eggs increased their risk for cardiovascular disease by 19 percent, and if those people already had diabetes, the risk for developing heart disease jumped to 83 percent with increased egg consumption.

New research published this year has shown that a byproduct of choline, a component that is particularly high in eggs, increases one's risk for a heart attack, stroke, and death.

Animal Protein

Inevitably, this discussion also leads to another question: "Even egg whites?" Yes, even egg whites are trouble. The reason most people purport to eat egg whites is also the reason they should be wary — egg whites are a very concentrated source of animal protein (remember, the raw material for all those yet-to-be-developed body parts?). Because most westerners get far more protein than they need, adding a concentrated source of it to the diet can increase the risk for kidney disease, kidney stones, and some types of cancer.

By avoiding eggs and consuming more plant-based foods, you will not only decrease your intake of cholesterol, saturated fat, and animal protein, but also increase your intake of protective fiber, antioxidants, and phytochemicals. Be smart! Skip the eggs and enjoy better healing.

Conclusion

There are reasonable arguments on both sides. I believe the forks over knives argument is stronger, but I decided to go with the moderate approach, I'll have hard boiled eggs occasionally or a veggie scramble but usually only once a week. I get filled, it tastes good, I have energy for the day, and I eat them in moderation. But that's just me. If you are diabetic or pre-diabetic, skip the eggs for sure. If not, make up your own mind, go with that and be happy and thankful. You'll be fine. Why did I go with eggs when I believe the argument is stronger on the no-egg side? Because my Aunt Ruthie, the nutritionist and my cousin Dr. Adam Fields who is the purest health enthusiast I've ever known . . . both said eggs were good for you and recommended eating them and I trust their judgement. My Aunt is 88 years old, still full of energy, she's beautiful and she eats eggs.

Dinner: Skip it if you can. About this time in my first week I wasn't that hungry. I know what you are thinking, *"Of course you weren't hungry, you didn't have anything tasty to eat."* Maybe, but mostly I was full of what my body needed for a change, so the hunger was satisfied. (Remember the principal, only eat when you are actually hungry and never because you are bored.) Because I was familiar with partial fasting (reread the fasting chapter) and I realized that I since I wasn't hungry, why not fast until the next morning, giving myself between 18 and 20 hours of stomach rest. In fact, sometimes not eating at all is as good or better then eating on schedule all the time. Giving your digestion system a chance to rest for a change is a good thing. It gets to catch up, heal, and restore itself. There were times during my first 6 weeks when I went a day and a half with no solid food, just water, kabocha and a smoothie. It's not that hard to do and this helps the body to revert to its normal weight for your size frame and bone structure. I lost 10 pounds in three weeks with no effort. The pounds just came off. I lost my belly and could get into my old jeans again and that was a bonus. I'm just saying, if you can go without a meal now and then, it won't hurt and, in fact, will help you reach your goal of vital health. The key here is, if you aren't hungry, don't eat and give your digestive system a needed rest.

Day 4.

Brunch (you skipped an early breakfast to extend your fast to 20 hours.)

Avocado slices on a bed of your favorite greens with your favorite oil-based dressing. Remember I like it easy and simple so I'm not making my own salad dressing to start with. To me buying a great tasting salad dressing is imperative. I know eating salads all the time can be boring but when you add an interesting tasting dressing, you have a new angle on eating healthy. I've tried a number of healthy store-bought dressings. Here are a few I recommend. Do yourself a favor and check these out. They will make eating leafy green vegetables way more interesting. They are excellent!

Favorite Healthy Store-Bought Dressings

Sometimes you simply don't have the time or inclination to make a dressing from scratch -and I totally get that - which is why I want to share my favorite healthy store-bought dressings with you. **I've gone all out here in the dressing department because I found it extremely helpful in enjoying salads, potatoes and various other dry foods.**

1. Whole Foods' Garlic Tahini Dressing
(Vegan, sugar-free, oil-free)

If I had to pick a favorite dressing this would probably be it. Tahini is the best and I love it combined with lemon and garlic for a zesty light dressing that's oil-free, low in calories and sugar, but still tastes rich. This is the dressing that Whole Foods uses for their garlicky kale salad. Ingredients: Filtered Water, Roasted Garlic Puree (Garlic, Citric Acid), Sesame Tahini (Ground Sesame Tahini (Ground Sesame Seeds), Apple Cider Vinegar, Soy Sauce (Water, Wheat, Soybeans, Salt, Alcohol (to retain freshness), Vinegar, Lactic Acid), Dried Yeast, Lemon Juice Concentrate, Non-GMO Corn Starch, Xanthan Gum.

- Nutrition: 2 Tablespoons = 45 cals, 2.5g fat, 96mg sodium, 4g carbs, 1g fiber, 0g sugar, 2g protein

2. Primal Kitchen Honey Mustard
(Gluten-free, dairy-free)

Being a honey mustard fan my whole life it's no surprise that this dressing from Primal Kitchen caught my eye immediately. After one taste I was hooked. I love the sweet and savory combo it's got going on. I love that Primal Kitchen dressings are made with avocado oil, which is loaded with antioxidants and omega-3 fatty acids.

- Ingredients: Avocado Oil, Water, Organic Apple Cider Vinegar, Organic Stone Ground Mustard (Water, Organic Mustard Seeds, Organic Vinegar, Sea Salt, Organic Spices), Organic Honey, Organic Lemon Juice Concentrate, Sea Salt
- Nutrition facts: 2 Tablespoons = 110 cals, 11g fat, 180mg sodium, 3g carbs, 0g fiber, 2g sugar, 0g protein

3. *Tessemae's Lemon Garlic*
(Vegan, gluten-free, sugar-free)

A tried and true, lemon and garlic together, is straight perfection. I love this as a simple dressing over kale or as marinade for chicken.

- Ingredients: Organic High Oleic Sunflower Oil, Organic Sunflower Oil, Organic Lemon Juice, Organic Extra Virgin Olive Oil, Organic Mustard (Organic Vinegar, Water, Organic Mustard Seed, Sea Salt, Organic Turmeric, Organic Spices), Organic Garlic, Sea Salt
- Nutrition facts: 1 Tablespoon, 90 cals, 10g fat, 105mg sodium, 0g carbs, 0g protein, 0g sugar, 0g protein

4. *Bragg's Vinaigrette*
(Gluten-free)

It's a simple vinaigrette, but loaded with flavor from the vinegar, liquid aminos, honey and spices. This is my go-to when I need a basic dressing to liven up a salad, but I also like using it as a marinade. And there are a few different flavors to mix it up.

- Ingredients: Bragg Organic Apple Cider Vinegar, Bragg Organic Extra Virgin Olive Oil, purified water, organic honey, organic garlic, Bragg Liquid Aminos, organic onion, organic black pepper, natural xanthan gum.
- Nutrition facts: 2 Tablespoons = 90 cals, 9g fat, 60mg sodium, 3g carbs, 0g fiber, 2g sugar, 0g protein

5. *Primal Kitchen Ranch*

(Gluten-free, sugar-free)

And for those "Ranch" lovers . . . Primal Kitchen is one of cleanest versions I've been able to find. Plus it tastes good. It makes a great dip for my <u>buffalo cauliflower wings</u> if you don't have time to make homemade ranch.

- Ingredients: Avocado Oil, Water, Organic Apple Cider Vinegar, Organic Distilled Vinegar, Cream of Tartar, Sea Salt, Gum Acacia, Organic Cage-Free Eggs, Organic Onion Powder, Organic Garlic Powder, Organic Lemon Juice Concentrate*, Nutritional Yeast, Konjac, Organic

Tapioca Starch, Organic Parsley, Organic Chives, Organic Dill, Organic Black Pepper, Organic Rosemary Extract.

- Nutrition facts: 2 Tablespoons = 140 cals, 15g fat, 210mg sodium, 2g carbs, 0g fiber, 0g sugar, 0g protein

6. Homemade Oil and Vinegar

(For the cooks and foodies — a genuine homemade recipe)

Oil and vinegar-based salad dressing, Thanks Gary and Ellen! Simple enough even for me.

2 parts red wine vinegar (the expensive kind)

1 part extra virgin olive oil (The best you can find)

Add fresh chopped garlic

Italian herbs

"Maille Mustard" ½ tsp.

Sugar ½ tsp , salt and fresh ground pepper to taste

Mix it all up in your favorite dressing bottle. Easy to make, easy to enjoy!

So, there you have 6 choices that will make eating leafy greens delicious and delightful. And because I believe this to be a real secret to eating all that green roughage, I'm going to list them all on the next page, together, so you can tear out the page, put the list in your wallet or purse right now and next time you go to the store you'll have the list handy.

Of course, you could copy the list and not tear out the page but I'm trying to make it as easy for you as possible. This can be a real key to your success.

Tear out this page

Here is the list: copy or tear out the page but try these dressings!

1. Whole Foods' Garlic Tahini Dressing (vegan, sugar-free, oil-free)
2. Primal Kitchen Honey Mustard (gluten-free, dairy-free)
3. Tessemae's Lemon Garlic (vegan, gluten-free, sugar-free)
4. Bragg's Vinaigrette (gluten-free)
5. Primal Kitchen Ranch (gluten-free, sugar-free)

Homemade oil-based salad dressing, Thanks Gary and Ellen! Simple enough even for me.

2 parts red wine vinegar (the expensive kind)

1 part extra virgin olive oil (The best you can find)

Add fresh chopped garlic

Italian herbs

"Maille Mustard" ½ tsp. – it's got to be Maille Mustard if possible.

Sugar ½ tsp , salt and fresh ground pepper to taste

Ok, I can't say enough about the importance of a tasty healthy dressing for your many salads . . . but I tried.

Day 4. (Continued)

Dinner: I treated myself to a piece of wild salmon on the 4th day. (Some people, vegans, will not choose to eat any flesh including fish but I'm not a Vegan . . . "not that there is anything wrong with that." (Seinfeld reference.)

I added quinoa heated up with some veggies. Very filling and satisfying meal. Now let's talk about the amazing food that quinoa is. Quinoa, pronounced "keen Wah" originated in Mexico and South America. My good friend Gary Nystrom went to Spain for three months and discovered quinoa and couldn't stop talking about it. His enthusiasm reminded me of the scene in the movie *Forest Gump* when his friend Bubba told him about the shrimp business. So many ways to serve it and enjoy it. The same applies to quinoa. Let's go deep into the world of quinoa.

"Quinoa is a good source of protein, fiber, iron, copper, thiamin and vitamin B6," said Kelly Toups, a registered dietician with the Whole Grains Council. It's also "an excellent source of magnesium, phosphorus, manganese and folate." Toups emphasized that "good source" means that one serving provides at least 10 percent of the daily value of that nutrient, while "excellent source" means that one serving provides at least 20 percent of the daily value of that nutrient.

A 2009 article in the *Journal of the Science of Food and Agriculture* stated that quinoa's "unusual composition and exceptional balance" of protein, oil and fat, as well as its minerals, fatty acids, antioxidants and vitamins, make it a highly nutritious food. The article also noted that phytohormones are found in quinoa, unlike many other plant foods. Phytohormones help regulate plant growth. Here are a few ways to enjoy quinoa.

1. Just plain — Quinoa has a lovely nutty flavor, and it can cook in less than 20 minutes, so I think quinoa makes a great substitute for pasta and rice.
2. As stuffing — We love the quinoa-stuffed dumpling .
3. Substituted for another grain, quinoa has a similar texture when cooked to other fine and fluffy whole grains like bulgur wheat.
4. In a grain salad — Quinoa is a fabulous base for easy, quick, filling grain salads.
5. Breakfast — Quinoa's high protein content and quick cooking time make it a great breakfast!

So, basically, quinoa goes with anything and everything and adds flavor and nutrition. They have it at grocery stores everywhere. Get this into your lifestyle. Again, if anything sounds interesting but you want more detail to go to our website to find my favorite cooking show videos. Thanks again You Tube! In today's world, there are no excuses for not knowing what or how to cook. It's all there, step by step procedures in how to make the healthy meal of your dreams. These people are geniuses. Learn a new recipe, enjoy the meal and experience brain plasticity!

Here are a few quinoa ideas that my friend Gary sent me, the guy who is the Bubba Gump for all things quinoa.

1. In a frying pan, sauté extra virgin olive oil, fresh garlic, onion, tomato, and spinach. Then add the quinoa and mix and enjoy. Make enough for leftovers.
2. Sauté garlic, onion, red bell peppers, in virgin olive oil add chopped tomatoes and tomato paste and or spaghetti sauce. Pour this sauce over a bed of cooked quinoa and enjoy. You can add a piece of salmon to add protein and satiety.
3. Try hot quinoa for breakfast with banana slices, blueberries almonds, walnuts etc. You can add a little almond milk to the mix if you like.

Day 5.

Breakfast: Avocado and Tomato salad. That's it, just slice up both and pour your favorite dressing on it and eat. You can skip the lettuce if you want, I do occasionally so I can enjoy more of the rich avocado taste. Yes, I love avocados. I didn't prefer them before I changed my lifestyle but when I heard how good they were for you I appreciated them more and now I love them . . . with the right dressing of course. Here is some food for thought about the goodness of the amazing avocado:

When it comes to nutrition, **avocados are in a class by themselves because** of the unusually large number of benefits they offer — more than 20, last count. Loaded with fiber, one avocado contains 36% of the daily requirement of vitamin K, 30% of the folate, and 20% each of the daily requirements of pantothenic acid (vitamin B5, needed to break down carbohydrates), vitamin B6, vitamin C, and potassium - more than twice the potassium of a banana. Vitamin E, niacin, and riboflavin levels deserve honorable mention. Eaten with other foods, your body is better able to absorb the nutrients, such as alpha- and beta-carotene and lutein.

Loosely described, lipids, their derivatives, and related substances are fatty acids. Scientists discovered only 40 years ago or so that they're not just simple building blocks, but perform complex, cell-regulating tasks on a molecular level, like messaging hormones, for example.

One study was undertaken to see if avocados might have more lipids than other fruits and vegetables, which, while rich in carotenoids, are lipid-challenged, impeding nutrient absorption. Researchers found that adding avocados to salad and salsa (foods used in the study) can significantly enhance your body's ability to take up the benefits of carotenoids, due primarily to the lipids in the avocados.[1]

The yellow-green color of avocados prompted another study, since color in other plant-based foods indicates carotenoid and other "bioactive" action, indicating possible cancer-fighting properties. The premise was that the monounsaturated fat in avocados might help your body absorb important bioactive carotenoids in combination with other fruits and vegetables, and therefore significantly reduce your risk of cancer.[2]

Avocado is one of the few fruits that will provide you with "good" fats. That means it can help keep your cholesterol levels in the healthy range and help lower your risk for heart disease.

So, you get the idea, avocados are awesome for you and it's wise to fall in love with them. They are almost a miracle food. They even use them in face creams, shampoos, and cosmetics. The Avocado is associated with "sophisticated health". It's a "cool and hip" food. Eat them! Health-style!

Lunch: Quinoa scramble with assorted veggies.

Dinner: Baked Sweet Potato or yam with cinnamon and raisins with a healthy dressing of your choice.

Day 6.

Breakfast: bowl of cereal with almond milk and fresh fruit. Now this can be tricky. You want a certain kind of cereal. Whole grains, not processed grains.

What we want is a Whole Food Plant Based Breakfast Cereal with Banana, Blueberries and Walnuts.

Ingredients

- 1/2 cup cooked cold millet 70g
- 1/2 cup cooked cold quinoa 70g
- 1/4 cup blueberries 20g
- 1/2 banana cut in slices
- 1/4 apple chopped
- 2 tablespoons chopped walnuts 10g
- 1 tablespoon maple syrup 15ml
- 1 cup fresh Almond Milk 235ml

I got this from Molly Patrick of Clean Food Dirty Girl. Check out her web site. Cleanfooddirtygirl.com Her company can be a big help in providing cooking and meal preparation ideas etc.

Lunch: Sliced hard-boiled eggs on a bed of spinach . . . with your favorite dressing.

Snack: Celery sticks and almond butter.

Dinner: Vegetable smoothie and a baked apple for desert.

Day 7.

Breakfast: bowl of fresh fruit. Note: Again, I shop at Costco because they have a lot of organic foods. I especially like their bags of frozen organic fruit, different kinds, quite a variety. I sometimes pour out a bowl full of the frozen berries and put them in the fridge in the evening and they are thawed out and ready to eat in the morning. Of course, you can just microwave the frozen berries and eat them. Your choice. I don't have a problem with the microwave oven, in fact I love them because they make cooking fast and easy, my style.

Lunch: Quinoa cooked in a pan with mushrooms and onions and spinach and olive oil.

Dinner: Ate my lunch leftovers. (Most of you will do a much better job of creating interesting meals than I have demonstrated here, but this worked for me.)

A hint: "Food batching". When you are making a special recipe make more than enough for one meal and freeze the leftovers and eat them when you feel like it later. Preparing food ahead of time, a few days in advance can be very helpful and is recommended.

More Helpful Hints

There will be times when you feel like eating something, but don't feel like making a meal. Or you are watching a food documentary on Netflix and you want to snack on something. I suggest that you always have some nuts on hand. Walnuts are one of the best and most nutrition-filled of all the nuts. Eating walnuts not only nourishes you but also the beneficial bacteria that live in your gut. This promotes the health of your gut and may help reduce disease risk. Almonds are good too. Nuts may reduce your risk of other chronic diseases. For example, eating nuts may improve blood sugar levels and lower your risk of certain cancers. Eating nuts may help reduce risk factors for many chronic diseases, including heart disease and diabetes. I'm snacking on almonds as I write this. Really fills you up.

In addition, I always have apples on hand. I wash them when I bring them home and put them in a bowl on my coffee table, so they are easy to get to and ready to eat. I eat them like a horse, or I'll slice them in quarters and sprinkle cinnamon on them, doesn't matter as long as you are eating them. Grapes are a great way to satisfy a sugar craving. Eat a bunch of grapes and you'll fill up and be satisfied sugar wise. So, in general, nuts and fruit will satisfy the need to put something into your mouth "right now" and make great healthy snacks. I like eating an apple while on a walk.

For you foodies - My favorite resource for Plant Based Cooking: Whole Food Plant Based Cooking Show with Jill www.plantbasedcookingshow.com and also check out www.cleanfooddirtygirl.com for detailed meal planning.

Chapter 18.

Believe in Yourself

During this process you have acquired wisdom and knowledge and you are "one" with your decision to become a healthy person and a health advocate in your immediate circle. The epiphany has taken root and the revelation is clear - you are ascending to a higher level of "being" and this is a good thing for everyone. If the goal of life is to strive to be the best we can be, which I contend that it is, then being the healthiest self is a great place to start.

And you, having made the decision, are stepping forward into the new and hopeful world of betterment and that starts with what you can control now — what's in your power today. You have knowingly taken a step in the right direction toward your best future self and that comes with the best outcomes and best experiences and, of course, we all want that. As humans we like the feeling of knowing we are doing the right thing, even if it's a little bit of a sacrifice. We do it for a good reason . . . it's not easy but we do it anyway . . . to materialize the best possible outcome.

Did you ever just want to start over and be someone else, someone who does the right thing always? Here's your chance! The Journey starts with a diet, a diet you decided on, to create the best possible you and you'll stick to the diet you choose because you researched it and it made the most sense to you. You are now in control of your health. You have reinvented yourself in a very positive way. You are in charge daily, keeping watch over unhealthy cravings and bringing forth strength and knowledge to quell the occasional attacks on your principals. You make the right decisions most of the time. You know what you are doing and why you are doing it and you do it most of the time (80 to 90 percent of the time). You aren't perfect yet, but you are working on it and you are "aware" of what you are eating every day. Better and improved health has suddenly materialized from your wise daily decisions.

You are expressing your inner power!

Again, everyone has the power within them to make the choice to be a heathy person. It starts with an understanding of why you are making the decision to change in the first place. Then the specific plan comes forth as a result of your own personal research that is easily found and totally available in books and on YouTube and on the web. (It's so easy now to learn anything you want. The tools of personal growth have

never been so readily available-take advantage of them).
You make a list of the food choices that *you* believe in and
you feel comfortable with based on your own research.
That is your starting diet. In the beginning you are
focused on sticking to the diet **one day at a time** just like a
reformed alcoholic makes it one day at a time.

You are smarter now. You can't un-see what you have
seen. You know too much now to go back to foolish bad
habits. You are no longer in the dark about this truth. Its
truth that leads to a better life . . . your better life. You are
your own informed nutritionist and you practice what you
preach. Soon, the days turn into weeks and you're still
focused on what's good for you despite an occasional
deviation. You notice that the hard decisions become
easier and easier. Before you know it, you are months into
this "living diet" that *you* created. You are happy now
because you are daily living a clean, righteous and healthy
lifestyle and lifestyles don't fail, they just are. You are on a
different path, the road less traveled. You've been (if you
will allow the term) born-again into this healthy lifestyle.
You are as you see yourself, you are becoming a new
healthy individual.

And, despite our progress, we need to be patient with those
who aren't there yet. Be an example but don't preach or
teach unless it's solicited or by example. I for one know
that unless you are ready, it's not going to happen. But be
healthy and be deliberate in what you put into your mouth
as you demonstrate a higher health-style experience. Be a
189

beautiful person inside and out. Be healthy and people will notice and be inspired.

As we said before, good health is achieved by being in balance. We want to eat a wide variety of nutritious foods. Fruits and Veggies, the more colorful, the better. Eat Organic when possible to avoid the potential pesticide residue you may consume on non-organic foods. Do this most of the time and you'll be healthy. But keep in mind, this is a journey of health and sometimes we get off the path and when we do, we know how to get back on the path because our inner compass always points us in the right direction. If you haven't reached a level of perfection yet, and few do, and If you find yourself at a Wedding or birthday party and are offered a piece of celebratory cake, and you want to partake, eat it and be thankful. We don't beat ourselves up about it. It's not going to kill you. Your body can withstand slights once in a while, just not a diet of them. (But beware of sugar, it's insidious.) We get knocked down, but we get up again! We never give up the quest, we are always striving to be our healthiest in every way. We are always positive about our adventurous journey to vibrant health.

Vibrant health doesn't happen overnight, it's a process. Just as a doctor is practicing medicine, we are practicing living the whole food, plant-based lifestyle. To review, the following is a short vision of what a whole food, plant-based lifestyle is. Know and understand it because this is your ultimate goal, your new lifestyle. This is the model that worked for me and is still working.

There is no clear definition of a what constitutes a whole-foods, plant-based lifestyle (WFPB diet). Remember, the WFPB diet is not necessarily a set diet — it's a lifestyle.

This is because plant-based diets can vary greatly depending on the extent to which a person includes animal products in their diet.

*Nonetheless, **<u>the basic principles of a whole-foods, plant-based lifestyle are as follows:</u>***

- *Emphasizes whole, minimally processed foods.*

- *Limits or avoids animal products.*

- *Focuses on plants, including vegetables, fruits, whole grains, legumes, seeds and nuts, which should make up the majority of what you eat.*

- *Excludes refined foods, like <u>added sugars</u>, white flour and processed oils.*

- *Pays special attention to food quality, with many proponents of the WFPB diet promoting locally sourced, organic food whenever possible.*

For these reasons, this diet is often confused with <u>vegan or vegetarian diets</u>. Yet although similar in some ways, these diets are not the same.

People who follow vegan diets abstain from consuming any animal products, including dairy, meat, poultry, seafood, eggs and honey. Vegetarians exclude all meat and poultry from their diets, but some vegetarians eat eggs, seafood or dairy.

The WFPB diet, on the other hand, is more flexible. Followers eat mostly plants, but animal products aren't off limits.

While one person following a WFPB diet may eat no animal products, another may eat small amounts of eggs, poultry, seafood, meat or dairy.

SUMMARY *The whole-foods, plant-based lifestyle emphasizes plant-based foods while minimizing animal products and processed items.*

Remember fellow travelers, this is not just a journey, it's an adventure! You'll be going to new and interesting places in your life. You'll be discovering how strong and resilient you really are. You'll open up to a whole new world of healthy and delicious foods and you'll make new health-foodie friends who are positive and interesting.

Don't wait another minute, **<u>Let The Adventure Begin! . . . Today!</u>**

One last inspirational thought brought to you by a fellow traveler, Molly Patrick, from "cleanfooddirtygirl.com"

You have one life in your beautiful, miraculous, delicious body . . .

So make it good.

Make it so good that you can feel your cells, alive and thriving, bringing your health and happiness with every single breath you take.

Make it rich.

So rich that when you go to bed at night, you can't wait to wake up in the morning.

Make it stunning.

So stunning that people don't look at you, they gaze at you, captivated by the energy and beauty that emanates from every pore of your being.

Make it inspiring.

So inspiring that your destination is an afterthought because you're so engrossed and smitten with the present moment.

Make it intentional.

So intentional that you break up with haphazardly scrambling and start a lifelong fling with time and space.

Make it mind-blowing.

So mind-blowing that you're able to do things that even your doctors told you couldn't be done.

Make it lovely.

So lovely that you admire and have a deep respect for every single one of your imperfections and feel at home and perfectly at ease in your beautiful body.

Make it empowered.

So empowered that you are responsible for every aspect of your gorgeous life and when you get off track, you appreciate the bump in the road, because there was a valuable lesson in the jolt.

Make it breathtaking.

So breathtaking that you inspire the people you love to make healthy choices in their own lives.

Make it magical.

So magical that you get exactly what you need, exactly when you need it, each and every time.

Make it easy.

So easy that the stuff you crave is exactly the stuff that supports you and makes you flourish.

This isn't a diet. This isn't a lifestyle. **This is your life!** You get one go around in the scrumptious vessel that is your body, and you have the power to live **EXACTLY** as you wish.

Take a breath and surrender to your happiness.

You are right where you need to be.

Join us in the revolt against ignorance. Join us on the path to enlightened eating. Be a part of the growing vanguard of aware and healthy

individuals as we change the world, one bite at a time. We are here to help!
<u>www.ourpassionforhealth.org</u>

Appendix

Top 10 Reasons to Pursue a Whole-food, Plant-based Lifestyle

Here are *my* top 10 reasons why choosing a wholefood plant-based lifestyle is a very good thing for you and your family. Feel free to add your own!

10. Philosophically, you are taking control of something that is most important to you and your future happiness. Eating right is one of the variables in life that you have total control over. No one else is to blame, no one else can stop you or even influence you once your mind is made up to go clean and healthy. You're in control and you are doing this, and it feels good in your body and soul.

9. You'll have more power. The decision, once made with understanding, gives you power. You made the decision, you're intelligently choosing what you feed yourself, your body is giving you positive feed-back, you're feeling better and feeling powerful because you are powerful.

8. You'll move up to a higher plane of vibration in your life. You've heard the expression, "That person has good vibes," right? The fact is, like almost everything in the universe, we are vibrating. We recognize people who put off good vibes and are repelled by bad vibes. Eating plants creates a whole healthy person and those people put off good vibes. You were able to break free from the masses and live on a higher plane, you'll feel different in a very good way, as each day is a little bit easier for you. Other people sense this in you and are drawn to your healthy "vibration".

7. You'll be a leader. Getting on board and being a part of the true health vanguard will show others that it's possible to break away. The best leaders lead by example and you'll be leading them.

6. You'll be a teacher. The best teachers teach by example. You'll be a good example of healthily living. People will ask you how you did it and you'll have a good and satisfying time giving them the knowledge and the answers that will be helpful to them on their path.

5. You'll be charismatic, and people will be drawn to you. When you make an obvious positive change in your life that is smart and healthy, people will be drawn to you and want to know your secret. When you are eating the food God put on the earth to nourish you, you'll create a vitality that people can see and feel and want to be around.

4. You will be happier. By making the choice to break away and do the right thing for yourself Healthwise, you'll feel that you are in control of your health and life and, in that, you are a success already, and that alone will make you a happier person.

3. You'll be living a meaningful life. Human beings have an inner desire to do something meaningful in their lives. (Check out "Maslow's Hierarchy of Needs".) Most people don't find themselves in a position to be that meaningful. Just by controlling what you put in your mouth and being an example for change with your own body (something everyone is capable of), you'll send out a positive healthy ripple effect to those all around you. In this way you will intrinsically be a meaningful person living a meaningful life.

2. You'll be changing the world in a good and positive way. For all the reasons above, you'll be a positive influence on your surroundings and by changing yourself, you'll be changing the world and making it a better place. Remember, everything good that you want to see in the world starts with you. "Let there be peace on earth and let it begin with me." Don't forget the song, *Man in the Mirror*.

1. The number one reason why eating right and getting healthy and taking control of your own health is one of the best ideas you could ever make is that you'll be healthy, free of illness and free of all physical suffering. You'll be vibrant, alert, energetic and have real inner strength, both for yourself and for your friends and family. Every living human being wants that! Don't you?

Additional Resources

My favorite plant-based "functional" doctors and experts on the subject who have books and You Tube videos I strongly recommend:

Dr. Alan Goldhamer, Dr. Joel Fuhrman, Dr. Michael Klaper, Dr. Doug Lyle, Dr. Colin T. Campbell, Dr. Caldwell Esselstyn, Dr. Michael Gregor, Jeff Novick NS

My favorite resource for Plant Based Cooking: Whole Food Plant Based Cooking Show with Jill

www.plantbasedcookingshow.com

Find more encouragement and motivation as well as additional resources and vision for America's health at the author's non-profit website:

www.OurPassionForHealth.org

About the Author and This Book

John Wilkins Spent the past 30 years in the financial services industry. He retired from "Wilkins Financial" in 2017 as his health began to deteriorate and moved from his home in Santa Cruz, California to Long Beach, Washington to be closer to his children and grandchildren. After experiencing the dramatic recovery of his health as described in this book, he formed "Our Passion For Health", a non-profit organization dedicated to public health education. "I spent most of my life helping rich people get richer…a profession that paid well but provided little personal satisfaction and was devoid of any social redeeming value. It turned out that getting sick was one of the best things that ever happened to me because it brought me to the revelation that resulted in finding a way to regain my health and gave me an opportunity to redirect my life toward something that is meaningful. I found the truth that can heal millions of suffering people just like me. I believe my message is profound and has the power to change lives for the better and that makes for a positive legacy."

To Thine Own Self Be True is John's first step in getting the message out that food can be one's medicine. His non-profit, "Our Passion For Health" is currently raising funds for the next project, a documentary entitled "Turning Back Time" about the importance of making one's health the number one priority in life and demonstrating the miraculous results of food as medicine. You can view the trailer at www.ourpassionforhealth.org

"The non-profit was named 'our' passion vs. 'my' passion because our goals are too big for any one person. It's going to take a lot of passionate partners to achieve what is possible…to turn the tide on the current American Health Crisis." Partner with John while creating your own meaningful legacy of health. To be a partner in this quest, contact John at:
john@ourpassionforhealth.org

www.ingramcontent.com/pod-product-compliance
Lightning Source LLC
Chambersburg PA
CBHW051443250726
48655CB00001B/214